RESTORE THE ROAR

RESTORE THE THE ROAR

PAT & KAREN SCHATZLINE

CHARISMA
HOUSE

Pat and Karen Schatzline's new book, *Restore the Roar*, will impose a moratorium on the paralyzing attacks of fear that have put your future on hold. The rhythm of every chapter stimulates great faith. This book will preach!

—JOHN KILPATRICK
PASTOR, CHURCH OF HIS PRESENCE

Pat and Karen Schatzline have done it again! They have taken a topic that is on the heart and mind of every person, including the church—fear—and strategically revealed key principles to help us walk in peace and power. Fear, rejection, and shame are no match for the message of the gospel! Through this powerful book Pat and Karen Schatzline reveal how you can abandon every insecurity and embrace a life of overcoming faith. We always enjoy having Pat and Karen as guests on Daystar Television as they speak into the lives of the lost, broken, and rejected on how to find hope and life-changing purpose through the power of the Word of God. Their latest work, *Restore the Roar*, is another great tool of encouragement for every believer! If you're ready to live courageously and walk in God-given authority, then *Restore the Roar* is a must-read!

—MARCUS AND JONI LAMB
FOUNDERS, DAYSTAR TELEVISION NETWORK

Pat and Karen Schatzline have created a powerful resource for all who have ever felt beaten down by dread, doubt, and disappointment. *Restore the Roar* is a call to arise and become the champion God created you to be.

—DANIEL KOLENDA
PRESIDENT AND CEO, CHRIST FOR ALL NATIONS

There is a sound rising up here on earth that is stronger and louder than the noise of this world. It is the sound that comes from the message of holy, pure men and women who announce with the testimony of their own lives the invincible power of the kingdom of God. Such are the lives of Pat and Karen, walking upon the waters of contrary circumstances and quieting the wind of fear. This book is for this moment in the history of the church of Jesus! The days in which we live declare that it is urgent that the shout of the people of God be heard. All creation, trapped in the silence of fear, awaits the manifestation of the sound of the sons of God! Thank you, Pat and Karen, for giving this present to our generation. Multitudes will be awakened by this book!

—APOSTLE MARCO A. PEIXOTO
FOUNDER AND PRESIDENT, CEIZS MINISTRIES

Restore the Roar is a bold and powerful book that will challenge and stir you. In this book Pat and Karen Schatzline shed light on the tactics of the enemy to keep you bound in fear, and they reveal to you the biblical formula for breaking fear and restoring your roar! This book will take you deeper in Him, break fear off your life, and awaken you to your identity and destiny.

—WARD SIMPSON
CEO, GOD TV

David ran to the roar of the Philistine. Courage is the premier quality needed to counter the ungodly challenges our society is roaring against us. Pat and Karen Schatzline are prophets and fearless speakers of truth against the roaring winds of darkness. Get on your armor. This book is going to move you from retreat to running to the roar!

—LARRY STOCKSTILL
PASTOR EMERITUS, BETHANY CHURCH

There is a breakthrough in store for you as you uncover God's Word and power through this book. May the courage of the Lion of Judah rise up in you and be released as you read these pages declaring the victory and authority God has for each of us.

—PHYLLIS SAWYER
CO PASTOR, CALVARY ASSEMBLY, DECATUR, ALABAMA

Fear is faith in the devil. Your desire to succeed must be greater than your fear of failure. Pat and Karen's powerful new book will restore the roar! It will cause you to slap yourself and say, "Not another day!" Get this book!

—GLEN BERTEAU
SENIOR PASTOR, THE HOUSE MODESTO

What an important and timely book! Fear is one of the enemy's most powerful weapons, yet very few books have been written that really show us how to overcome our fears. And so many believers have lost their confidence, their authority, their trust, their faith. That's why I'm so glad Pat and Karen Schatzline have written *Restore the Roar*, sharing their own struggles with fear—and the path to victory in Jesus. Your roar will be restored as you read and act!

—DR. MICHAEL L. BROWN
HOST, *THE LINE OF FIRE*
AUTHOR, *JEZEBEL'S WAR WITH AMERICA*

They nailed it! Once again revivalists Pat and Karen Schatzline capture the heart of the Father for His children in this timely message for the church. As the people of God read this book, a powerful roar will be heard rising from a slumbering church that will bring the kingdom to earth. For far too long the enemy has silenced the church in ignorance and lack. No more! Arise, church, and sound the roar! This is a must-read for every believer and especially every church leader.

—TODD SMITH
SENIOR PASTOR, CHRIST FELLOWSHIP CHURCH

It takes men and women of a certain caliber to stand up, especially in the midst of a hostile crowd, and speak the truth. There are not many who will do this and risk everything. But in every generation God reserves for Himself those like John the Baptist, who in the face of extreme opposition will thunder the righteousness of God and give the call to repent. The story is told of a man who came to hurt George Whitefield, that British fire-brand preacher, because he was offended by something White-field said. The man told the preacher, "I came here to hear you with my pocketful of stones intending to break your head; but your sermon got the better of me, and broke my heart." This book, *Restore the Roar*, will put spine in your backbone. Both Pat and Karen have modeled this for us and led the way.

—YANG TUCK YOONG
SENIOR PASTOR, CORNERSTONE COMMUNITY CHURCH

Pat and Karen Schatzline have written a book that is nothing less than a declaration of war on the spirit of fear. *Restore the Roar* is a road map, leading the reader to peace, renewed power, and victory in Jesus.

—JIM RALEY
PASTOR, CALVARY CHRISTIAN CENTER

It is often during the darkest times in life that the greatest revelation is birthed. It is during those times that if we let Him, God will come close and reveal Himself to us in new ways. Pat and Karen share with great transparency the difficult times in their lives, and with great clarity and deep insight they offer the revelation God gave them while they were going through those times. We all go through hard times. We all lose our courage. We all stand insecure and fearful at times. This phenomenal book will lift you, encourage you, and strengthen you. It will indeed cause you to rise up with new confidence and restore *your* roar.

—BISHOP DAVID AND PASTOR KATHIE THOMAS
VICTORY CHRISTIAN CENTER

We who believe in Christ are part of a new creation generation born into a world that is wallowing in gross darkness. It is the divine mandate of teachers to equip today's saints to overcome. In this book Pat and Karen provide practical and spiritual keys, shrouded in compassion and loving faith, that indeed empower believers to emerge free of fear and insecurities. As you read, your spirit will be strengthened and emboldened with supernatural courage!

—FRANK AMEDIA
FOUNDER AND CHAIRMAN, POTUS SHIELD COUNCIL
FOUNDER, TOUCH HEAVEN MINISTRIES

Pat and Karen Schatzline have a prophetic mandate to see this generation set free from fear. Every page of *Restore the Roar* will encourage and equip you to walk into the future God has for your life.

—AARON BURKE
PASTOR, RADIANT CHURCH

When you've been in a place where you've heard the voice of fear, it's only then that you realize the power of the roar. Pat and Karen's own battle with the enemy of their faith has allowed them to share how we too can release the power God has put within us to press through and declare victory. My takeaway is this: our battles are manifested in the natural world, but it's through the roar that the supernatural is released to give us the win. Pat and Karen remind us that we were never promised a fearless life—only that we can be fearless in the face of it.

—STEVE ALESSI
PASTOR, METRO LIFE CHURCH

I've read only a handful of books outside of the Bible that are infused with enough of God's presence to make me shake and weep. This book is one of them. This isn't just another book on the subject of fear. It's a divine blast of the Holy Spirit to set us free!

—CHRIS PHILLIPS
PASTOR, RIVER OF LIFE CHURCH

Wow! I love this book! Pat and Karen have written an inspiring book that will provide you with insights to properly deal with the enemy called fear that would attempt to defy your trust in the One who is your provider, protector, and perfecter. Lift up your voice and shout to God. He will be your strength and your song. Let the rock of your salvation teach you how to stand in the invincible place where you are strong in the Lord and the power of His might.

—Dr. Mark Spitsbergen
Pastor, Abiding Place

In their great book *Restore the Roar* Pat and Karen remind us that God has a plan to defeat Satan and his use of fear to try to stop us from accomplishing God's purposes in our lives. The truths in this book have stirred my passion for the enemy's defeat. If you read *Restore the Roar*, I know it will fill you with the same passion.

—Carl Stephens
Pastor, Faith Assembly

Visit the author's website at https://raisetheremnant.com and http://SchatzlineBooks.com.

Library of Congress Cataloging-in-Publication Data

Names: Schatzline, Pat, author.
Title: Restore the roar / by Pat and Karen Schatzline.
Description: Lake Mary, Florida : Charisma House, 2019.
Identifiers: LCCN 2019016860 (print) | LCCN 2019980635 (ebook) | ISBN
    9781629996554 (trade paper) | ISBN 9781629996561 (ebook)
Subjects: LCSH: Fear--Religious aspects--Christianity. | Trust in
    God--Christianity. | Spiritual warfare.
Classification: LCC BV4908.5 .S344 2019 (print) | LCC BV4908.5 (ebook) |
    DDC 248.8/6--dc23
LC record available at https://lccn.loc.gov/2019016860
LC ebook record available at https://lccn.loc.gov/2019980635

19 20 21 22 23 — 9 8 7 6 5 4 3 2
Printed in the United States of America

DEDICATION

THIS BOOK IS dedicated to our amazing children, Abby, Nate, and Adrienne, along with our beautiful grandchildren, Jack and Andy, and every generation to come thereafter. You make us so proud. You make us want to continually strive for a deeper walk with God. You are our why, and you own our hearts. It is for each of you that we fight to break every stronghold of fear off our family. It is for you that we will always push past fear, pain, disappointments, obstacles, and struggles. It is for you that we will always rise above the changing tides of culture. It is for you that we will walk in faith, always trusting God in all things and in every season of life.

We challenge you to always press forward and never allow the enemy to cause you to think you are less than or that you cannot be a voice of hope and freedom to your generation. You were created for a purpose. You were created for something bigger than yourself. Your voice matters. Never shrink back, never hide in the shadows, and never listen to the voice of fear and insecurity. You are worthy, you are capable, and you are destined to overcome obstacles and walk in victory. You are champions and will do great and mighty exploits for God.

This journey with God will always be a great big, amazing adventure. Embrace every part of the journey with passion, purpose, boldness, and courage. Be fierce in your pursuit of God's presence. Always have ears to listen for His voice, and He will speak to you. Know that you are a powerful force against darkness when you know who God has called you to be. Dad and Mom love you with all our hearts.

We also dedicate this book to every person who has felt overwhelmed, insecure, inadequate, unworthy, and backed into a corner by the enemy. We want you to know that you have permission to step out and be bold and courageous. We want you to know that God wants you to walk in power, love, and a sound mind that cannot be affected by the schemes of the enemy. It is time to wake up, rise up, and be the one who puts the enemy on the run.

Generations to come will be rescued and revived by your courage. You were not created for fear. You were created for victory. No more fear!

CONTENTS

Foreword by Sid Roth xvii

Foreword by Al and Tava Brice xix

Introduction: We Were Afraid to Write
This Book xxiii

1. Restore the Roar 1

2. Do You Trust Me? 11

3. The Formula for Defeating Fear 27

4. When the Shadow Looms 39

5. Just Breathe 55

6. Courage, It's Me! 67

7. Peace in the Storm 85

8. Let Your Praise Be Louder Than Your Fear 103

9. The Hidden 123

10. Don't Give Up; Get Moving! 135

11. Have Your Day in Court 151

12. This Is Your Now 173

13. If They Can, We Can 195

Appendix 207

Notes 211

About the Authors 217

FOREWORD

WHEN I WAS a Jewish nonbeliever in Jesus, I not only experienced normal fear as a sinner but also demonic fear with no answers! At age twenty-nine I went searching for happiness. I left my wife, young daughter, and career-type job, searching for happiness. The only problem was I didn't know its address! I took a New Age meditation course and learned how to lower my consciousness and invite an imaginary friend inside of me. This friend would answer any question, even about the future. But when I was in too deep, I realized this "friend" was evil—a demon in fact. If you know the story of *The Exorcist*, I lived it! As a Jew I looked everywhere but to Jesus for help, not knowing He was the *only* power stronger than the demon.

I was sinking for the third and final time in the ocean with no help. A Christian friend said if I asked Jesus for help, He would rescue me because Jesus' power was greater than the devil's power. I would not consider this option as a Jew. But when you are sinking with no help, you will grab whatever rope is thrown to help you.

I went to bed on the worst night of my life. I didn't want to die, but life was too hard. The fear was so strong I knew that if Jesus, my last hope, didn't help, I didn't want to live and face this fear anymore! But my hero rescued me. I experienced the peace of God when what I now know was His glory entered my bedroom. The glory overwhelmed the fear! The demon could not take the glory of God.

I knew it was Jesus, my Messiah, who had rescued me. Then God spoke to me and quoted the Jewish prophet Malachi. At the time, I didn't even know what I heard was in the Bible. He said, "I hate divorce. Return to your wife and daughter." God restored my family, my mind, and my future. I have now walked with God for over forty-eight years. I have been married to the wife of my youth for fifty-five years. And I still live in the salvation glory that rescued me.

But the fear came back as a new believer in Jesus with a vengeance. It tried to take advantage of my ignorance of the Bible. I wish I would have had the Schatzlines' book so I would have learned to roar like a lion over the enemy. I had to learn these principles the hard way, but fortunately others won't have to do the same. This generation will need to overcome the same or even worse demons than I dealt with. You will need to know this revelation that God has downloaded to the Schatzlines for such a time as this. Get ready to roar!

—Sid Israel Roth
Host, *It's Supernatural!*

FOREWORD

REMNANT CRUSADERS PAT and Karen Schatzline are resolute prophetic voices for our time. We have personally observed the genuineness of their faith throughout two decades of friendship and ministry networking. Year after year they faithfully stewarded revival encounters and revolutionary books to youth, and then they broadened the scope of their ministries to the entire family of God. Their kingdom passion is no dying ember nor even a steady burn; rather they continually kindle their internal flames, resulting in an ever-increasing, all-consuming blaze of God's glory. Their book *Restore the Roar* is their next firestorm postured to consume every hungry heart in its path.

The first recorded words Adam uttered after sin came into the world included "I was afraid" (Gen. 3:10). When the angel spoke to Mary and told her she would give birth to Jesus, he said, "Do not be afraid" (Luke 1:30). When Jesus appeared to His disciples after purchasing our salvation on the cross, He told them, "Do not be afraid" (Matt. 28:10). The only answer to fear is faith and love, as 1 John 4:18 says: "There is no fear in love; but perfect love casts out fear, because fear involves torment. But he who fears has not been made perfect in love" (NKJV).

As pastors and fellow ministers we are observing in people a deep desire to fulfill their God-given destinies. They truly want to be successful and make a difference for the kingdom of God. There is, however, a hidden X factor, a mountain of darkness that rises up to halt every endeavor of faith. It bellows at each one of us and defies us to really believe that God is going to do everything He promised us. This debilitating roar comes from the spirit of fear, which is the most effective weapon the kingdom of darkness possesses.

Fear is the energy of the domain of darkness. Through it Satan keeps multitudes in a mental state of slavery. Even though as Christians we possess a far superior power and authority, we allow these tormenting thoughts, anxieties, and worries to erase our faith in God's provision. In *Restore the Roar* Pat and Karen have called this X factor out onto the battlefield.

The uniqueness of this work lies in the unified voices of both a mother and father in the faith. Though both of the Schatzlines minister powerfully as individuals, they recognize God beckoning them to minister as one. Today's generation craves the impartation that only healthy spiritual parents can provide.

Pat presents the visionary, provocative clarion call of the Father to reach the world with His love. He instructs

God's sons and daughters with Scripture and practical strategies for fully achieving heaven's mandate. He trumpets the battle roar to cast off strongholds of fear and to prevail against darkness to God's glory. He faithfully conveys to readers the Father's blessing, which says, "You are enough because you are Mine!"

Karen's voice is that of a mother. Her words are like a lullaby that soothes the fears of the heart with the palpable love of the Holy Spirit. She holds up the mirror of God's Word, reflecting the image of Christ within readers so they are securely grounded when Satan breathes threats and condemnation. Karen directs sons and daughters into paths of righteousness with candor and clarity for the glory of God.

The Holy Spirit has given Pat and Karen Schatzline a divine revelation to defeat fear—once and for all. Their unified voices will propel you into a greater realm of faith and confidence. Get ready to roar and soar into your God-given destiny.

—PASTOR AL AND TAVA BRICE
COVENANT LOVE CHURCH

WE WERE AFRAID TO
WRITE THIS BOOK

W E ARE LIVING in a day and age when fear rules the lives of believers and nonbelievers alike. From terrorist attacks to man-made disasters and natural disasters, many are glued to the twenty-four-hour cycle of nonstop bad news, battling at every level with insecurities, fear of failure, and even fear of stepping into what God has for them.

Consider this definition the Lord gave us:

> Fear is the thief of yesterday's dream,
> the intimidator of today's promises, the
> decapitator of headship, the emasculator
> of tomorrow's warriors, the cage of God's
> eagles, and the enemy's greatest weapon to
> hold us hostage.

Fear is the greatest threat that exists to believers. Yet fear is nothing more than a straw man of the enemy. It is a learned or perceived aberration that grows into an absolute.

The opposite of fear is peace. The title given to Jesus in Isaiah 9:6 is "Prince of Peace"! We have a promise in our Savior and in Scripture that tells us God's peace will crush Satan (Rom. 16:20). Satan desires to steal both the very title bestowed upon Jesus and the DNA of our salvation. Through fear he will try to ravage our souls and cause us to disappear from the places God has for us to stand strong in and occupy. When the Spirit of God removes the spiritual blinders from our eyes and exposes the enemy's fear tactics, we are able to stand strong with the weapons of peace. The Bible tells us, "And the peace of God, which transcends all understanding, will guard your hearts and your minds in Christ Jesus" (Phil. 4:7). We need to understand that God has an answer and a recipe to set us free from fear and lead us into a place of peace, destiny, and purpose.

There was a point at which fear tried to overtake us and keep us from writing this book. We knew this message had to go out, but we also understood there is always a battle when you confront the lies of the enemy because he hates to be exposed. We have learned that whatever you choose to write about or crusade against in the Spirit will inevitably try to take you out. It began in the fall of 2018 when the very thing we were going to confront decided to knock once again at our front door. We had just met with our dear friends and publishers of many years at Charisma Media. During the meeting we shared all that God had done in our lives over the last few months, including the details of our greatest battle and our desire to write this book in response. Their response was an absolute and resolute, *"Write the book!"* Nevertheless, two days after agreeing to write this book, I (Pat) began to have some concerns. We were exhausted from the battle we had just been through, and I began to wonder if we had both been too excited to share how God had radically healed her and how we had overcome the greatest battle of our lives. We knew this message would be a black eye to the enemy. Yet I also knew that in the process of writing this book, I would have to confront the issue of fear that had a hold on me my entire life.

For many years I would have nightmares of plane crashes or my family facing terrible tragedy. Most often these dreams took place when I traveled, only hours before I would be walking on stage to minister. I understand what Solomon meant when he wrote in Ecclesiastes 5:3, "A dream comes when there are many cares." Those nightmares often came just before some of the most powerful moves of God we have ever seen. Over the years those troubling dreams had dissipated. In fact I never remember having a nightmare while at home until we chose to write this book. As the enemy began to attack me in the night hours, I wasn't sure I was ready to resume this war. While I wrestled with my fears, Karen responded with faith.

"Pat," she said, "it is time to confront the enemy of our past, present, and future. This book will restore so many and equip them to live once again. Satan is the one who is afraid. He knows that if people get free from fear, they will be able to do the impossible. They will rise up and take back what has been stolen by the lie of fear."

I knew immediately that she was right. Faith and courage began to rise in me. How dare Satan try to intimidate me! I called my dad and shared the battle. He said, "Son, before you go to sleep each night, simply purge the atmosphere. Rebuke the enemy in your home or hotel room, then watch what happens." His words rang true in my heart. We had done this when we brought our daughter home from China and she was having night terrors. Immediately I began to pray and rebuke the nightmares before I went to sleep at night, and the dreams subsided.

WAKE UP, SLEEPER!

> That is why it is said: "Wake up, sleeper, rise from
> the dead, and Christ will shine on you."
> —EPHESIANS 5:14

Because we decided to move forward with this book, our goal is to make Satan pay back what he has stolen in your life and in our lives. The enemy is not concerned about who we have been but where we are going. He wants to overwhelm us with fear. For far too many believers there is a battle raging. It is time to take back our territory! It is time to conquer fear! We intend this to be a supernatural handbook on defeating fear and arising and being courageous. It is the desire of our hearts that this book awaken all believers to walk in their God-given authority. Together we can defeat the lies of the enemy. In the chapters that follow, you will learn what it means to restore the roar and receive the very breath of God and the freedom to trust the Father. You will learn how fear is the embryo of courage. In fact you must first be afraid in order to find your courage!

Every believer has been given the "God tools" to win in the battlefield of the mind and destroy the illusions from the enemy. We must always remember we will never lose what we have entrusted to God's loving care and protection. The psalmist spoke correctly when he wrote in Psalm 56:3, "In the day when I am afraid, I will trust in You" (MEV). Fear is just a distraction of the enemy, not our final destination. God is still in charge! He can deliver us!

We are promised in His Word that regardless of what we face, He is there with us. "I sought the LORD, and he answered me; he delivered me from all my fears" (Ps. 34:4). As you journey with us through this book, you might just find out that your day of hiding under the bedcovers is over because "God has not given [you] a spirit of fear, but of power and of love and of a sound mind" (2 Tim. 1:7, NKJV). It is time to arrest the lies of the enemy and restore the roar in God's lions. Proverbs 28:1 says, "The wicked run away when no one is chasing them, but the godly are as bold as lions" (NLT). Are you ready to roar, to take your rightful place in the kingdom of God? The first step in that direction is to defeat the spirit of fear.

—PAT AND KAREN SCHATZLINE

P.S. While you are reading this handbook of hope, stop periodically and listen. You might just hear a roar from the heavenlies coming from the Lion of the tribe of Judah!

OUR PRAYER FOR YOU

Dear God, we praise You for being our waymaker and peace provider. Lord, all of us reading this book are very special to Your heart. You have

heard our cries, felt our pain, and brought com-
fort in times of mourning. You have never left
our side. You, O Lord, even know our darkest
secrets and our deepest fears. You have prom-
ised to never leave us or forsake us. We pray that
this book brings healing, hope, refreshment, and
boldness to help every reader withstand the lies
of Satan. We declare that this day from our very
gut a roar of victory is arising. You need all of us,
Lord, to take our rightful place in Your kingdom.
Our voices of truth are needed to denounce the
lies of culture, restore the place of encounter in
the church, and bring hope where others are lost.
God, may this book restore to us the weapons to
defeat fear once and for all. Amen.

Now, let's go get your roar back.

CHAPTER 1

RESTORE THE ROAR

The lion has roared—who will not fear? The Sovereign
LORD has spoken—who can but prophesy?

—AMOS 3:8

THERE HAS NEVER been a better time in history for the righteous to speak up and stand their ground. We are at a crossroads all around the world where declaring biblical truth is considered hate speech and tolerance is a belief in nothing. The greatest enemy of truth is silence. Satan knows that if he can take your voice, then you are no longer a threat. You may have heard the quote, "The only thing necessary for the triumph of evil is for good men to do nothing."[1] I (Pat) must confess that after years of ministry all over the world, there are times when I feel as though my voice has grown weary. I often desire a season of peace and quiet amid the chaos, to escape the battle.

Weariness and exhaustion have the ability to not only quiet the dream but also silence the messenger. If we are not careful, weariness can cause us to go into hiding rather than into a place of rest. The enemy will always try

1

to steal our voices with intimidation, frustration, trials, and tribulation. Warrior saints are handicapped when we allow ourselves to become victims because we forget God has already won the war. My heart's cry is "O dear God, that we never mistake lethargy as peace."

In September 2018 I was in a hotel room in Pennsylvania. It was very early in the morning. I had spoken the night before at a conference in Scranton, and God had moved mightily. This was during the time the United States was deeply embroiled in a battle for the confirmation of a conservative Supreme Court justice. It was actually more than a battle. It was an all-out war. The twenty-four-hour news cycle and social media were lit with the issue. From all accounts of friends and colleagues the candidate was actually a very good man. This particular judge was a constitutional conservative with biblical values. Horrified, I watched as a man of upstanding character was devoured by the liberal media with unsubstantiated claims against his character. He and his family were being publicly lynched on a daily basis. The fact of the matter was that this man was a pro-life justice. That was truly his greatest crime. If approved, he could change the balance of the courts regarding *Roe v. Wade* and other conservative issues. The sacred cow of the secular Left is to maintain access to abortion. If approved, this justice could tip the balance on the court to overturn *Roe v. Wade*.

I had decided that due to the media hype and strong feelings on each side I would remain quiet, forgetting that if we are not careful, the radical voices of perversion will only grow louder as we grow ever more silent out of fear.

There were plenty of days when I said to myself, "Why even speak up?" After all, most of the leaders of the church were deathly silent about the issue. The sad reality is that when the church and shepherds remain silent when they should speak up, the innocent suffer. That is exactly how Hitler rose to power in Germany.

As the onslaught continued, I reminded myself to stay in my lane. "Why invite the haters?" I asked myself. Truth be known, we all have an innate desire to be loved, cheered, and appreciated, including me. The best way to build a following is to just stay out of the battle. Then everyone will give you a nod of approval.

I once heard it said, "Monuments are never built for those who criticize but for those who ignored the critics." In all honesty, I was not speaking up because I was afraid. Karen and I had just survived the greatest battle of our lives, and fear was crippling me. I understand Psalm 55:4–6, which says, "My insides are turned inside out; specters of death have me down. I shake with fear, I shudder from head to foot. 'Who will give me wings,' I ask—'wings like a dove?'" (MSG). Those verses describe where I was. Everything within me wanted to cry out, "God, get me out of here on dove's wings. I want some peace and quiet. I want a walk in the country. I want a cabin in the woods. I'm desperate for a change from rage and stormy weather."

Nowadays we are taught that people do not want to hear a message of change but rather a message of hope. In other words, don't tell me how to live; instead tell me how well I am doing at living. It is a whole lot easier to preach a hyped-up message of victory layered with some well-timed shouting and clapping than a message of repentance that challenges us to draw near to God. However, that is not what burns in our hearts. Karen and I burn with a message of awakening, a "yet even now" message. The prophet Joel declared, "'Yet even now,' declares the LORD, 'return to me with all your heart, with fasting, with weeping, and with mourning'" (Joel 2:12, ESV).

This type of message is not always relevant or welcome in our churches. We are living at a time when it is much easier to feed the flock with cotton candy that has no nutritional value than to preach a life-giving, meat-filled message of truth. It is much easier to keep the masses happy with self-help messages that do not limit personal freedom or invoke conviction. I have found that a message from the pulpit declaring holiness, truth, and freedom is not usually on the menu of most churches. We have heard time and again that many mainstream leaders consider the message of the restoration of the altar to be a concept that works only in a retreat or private prayer setting. I know this is not true. We have personally seen hundreds of thousands meet God at the altar and find freedom, hope, and salvation when we share this message. Nevertheless it can get very weary carrying a message like this. Just when Karen and I think it is time to step away from ministry for a while, we hear His voice—the voice of Jesus awakening these two wandering saints to once again stare at the cross of redemption. He will often whisper into the stillness of our night to remind us that He hasn't gone anywhere.

DEEP CALLS TO DEEP

Likewise God is eager to awaken you once again to go deep in Him. "Deep calls to deep at the noise of Your waterfalls; all Your waves and Your billows passed over me. Yet the LORD will command His lovingkindness in the daytime, and in the night His song will be with me, a prayer to the God of my life" (Ps. 42:7–8, MEV). I believe that if we ignore the "deep calls to deep" moments, we will soon believe the shallow end of the pool is deep. If you want to go deep, take off the floaties and dive in where you cannot stand up on your own. I must warn you though that when you try to go deep in God, someone will always try to throw you a rope called *settling*. You cannot settle in the depth of God.

I have learned the longer you are away from the place of encounter with God, the more satisfied you become with being normal according to the world's standards. In fact it is much like what happened to the prophet Elijah when he ran into the cave in fear for his life. God said to him, "Why are you here, Elijah?" (1 Kings 19:9, MEV). Remember, Jezebel had threatened Elijah after he killed the prophets of Baal, telling him through one of her servants, "So let the gods do to me and more also, if I do not make your life as the life of one of them by tomorrow about this time" (1 Kings 19:2, MEV). Elijah ran for his life and was now hiding in a cave. God was not really asking him, What are you doing here? Rather, He was reminding him of his mission. Leonard Ravenhill once said, "A man who is intimate with God is never intimidated by man."[2] We must no longer be intimidated by man or accusations or threats.

5

Early that morning in the hotel room in Pennsylvania, I was awakened by the voice of the Lord. He said to me, "Pat, where did your roar go? Where is the roar of My lions?" Startled, I sat up in bed and immediately began to pray. The whisper of God had shaken me to the core, bringing to mind one of my favorite verses in the Bible, Matthew 10:27: "What I tell you in the dark, speak in the daylight; what is whispered in your ear, proclaim from the roofs." God will often whisper a message to you that eventually becomes a public proclamation. This was one of those times.

The Lord went on to say to me, "My people are perishing for lack of knowledge. They have lost their will to fight. Fear, exhaustion, and culture have taken their roar away. They must be awakened and realize they are called to be voices of truth that carry freedom in their hearts and fire in their spirits. Restore the roar! Tell My lions to roar once again!"

I must admit I was perplexed and confused, and I began to weep before the Lord. In fact I stood in my hotel room that day, praying and crying out for over an hour with the realization that I too had become quiet. One of my heroes, Salvation Army general William Booth, said, "We must wake ourselves up! Or somebody else will take our place, and bear our cross, and thereby rob us of our crown."[3] We must take the message of 1 Corinthians 16:13–14 and make it our marching orders: "Keep your eyes open, hold tight to your convictions, give it all you've got, be resolute, and love without stopping" (MSG).

Karen and I had just spent a year in fear. The battle had been intense. Just as a parent awakens a child from sleep to get ready for school or a teacher raps a ruler on your desk to end a daydream, God was saying, "Wake up, Pat! Your mission is not over. Put your armor on once again and enter the fight." I had been wandering a bit aimlessly since our battle, and God was calling me back to the field. Many who are reading this book right now wear nothing but the helmet of salvation. The Bible tells us that God has a whole suit of armor for us. (See Ephesians 6:10–18.) He provides all we need for any battle we face. We just need to equip ourselves.

RELEASE YOUR ROAR!

With God's word ringing in my heart, I immediately began to search the Scriptures concerning lions. Proverbs 28:1 says, "The wicked run away when no one is chasing them, but the godly are as bold as lions" (NLT). Did you hear that? We are called to be bold as lions! You and I are called to roar! Regardless of how exhausted and weary we become, we must seek the Lord once again. We must once again take our rightful place of authority. And when we do, God will provide what we need for the battle. "The lions may grow weak and hungry, but those who seek the LORD lack no good thing" (Ps. 34:10).

I believe the Lord is saying the restoration of the roar is when His Spirit arises once again from the depths of our bellies, where the roar has been caged under lock and key by low expectations, wounded spirits, and lack of hunger. He desires to awaken our prophetic voices once more. Just look at Amos 3:8: "The lion has roared—who will not fear? The Sovereign LORD has spoken—who can but prophesy?"

If you've ever been on the savanna, you know that the roar of a lion momentarily stops everything in its tracks. The voice of God will do the same in your life. In fact it will do more. It will awaken your prophetic voice. Just as the roar of the lion brings fear for one's well-being, the voice of the prophet should restore the fear of the Lord.

As I pressed in further regarding lions, Holy Spirit began to reveal things to me. Did you know that "lions roar to tell other lions where they are, to show how big they are and to warn lions from other prides to keep away from their home territory"? Lions "do this mostly just before sunrise and [around] sunset when they are most active."[4] Did you catch those three aspects of a lion's roar? Let's look at each individually.

First, a lion's roar is to let other lions know where his territory is. Lions are at the top of the food chain and are fearsome hunters. The Bible likens Satan to a lion on the prowl. First Peter 5:8 says, "Be alert and of sober mind. Your enemy the devil prowls around like a roaring lion looking for someone to devour." The devil is a prowler, and we are called to be aware of his schemes (2 Cor. 2:11). He loves to hunt big game, and his target is believers. He wants to make you a trophy above his fireplace. It is time let him know you are not his prey. If the enemy invaded your territory or took land from you, then it is time to put him on notice. It is time to release your roar!

A lion's roar can also indicate how big it is. Proverbs 30:30 characterizes lions as the "mightiest among beasts and does not turn back before any" (ESV). We must not forget who we are and whose we are. We are "children of

God" (John 1:12). That's right! We have birthright status. Not only that, but according to 2 Corinthians 5:21, we are the "righteousness of God." Jesus is our righteous Lion! Revelation 5:5 says, "And one of the elders saith unto me, Weep not: behold, the Lion of the tribe of Judah, the Root of David, hath prevailed to open the book, and to loose the seven seals thereof" (KJV). God is telling us that the story of mankind ends well. Our Lion wins!

We were created to overthrow the kingdom of darkness. The prophet Amos put it this way: "Does a lion roar in the forest if there's no carcass to devour? Does a young lion growl with pleasure if he hasn't caught his supper?" (Amos 3:4, MSG). I truly believe there is a supernatural shift taking place in the kingdom of God. Those who have lived in fear are beginning to realize they are God's lions. They are engaging in the battle once again because the need for fierce warriors is great. Your family, your friends, and your city need you back in the battle. Let your roar, your declaration of victory, be heard in the land!

A third trait of lions is that while they roar at various times during the day, their roaring typically reaches a peak around sunset and just before sunrise. Notice that the lion's loudest roars can be heard twice a day. What if the same could be said of you? Psalm 92:1–2 says, "It is good to praise the LORD and make music to your name, O Most High, proclaiming your love in the morning and your faithfulness at night." The Bible says the fire of the altar is to be lit morning and night. (See Ezra 3, especially verse 3.) Imagine what would happen if you spent mornings and evenings in prayer. You would get your faith back! Remember, Jesus "is called

Faithful and True" (Rev. 19:11). I like to say, "In the morning Jesus is faithful, and by evening He has proven to be true."

God is calling us to reclaim the land, declare our true identities, and offer praise to Jesus in the morning and the evening. If you will follow these simple steps, then you will divorce fear and stand once again on the rock. Faith will arise and answer the door when the enemy knocks. A dear friend once shared with me a quote he read in an old bed-and-breakfast in Ireland: "Fear knocked at the door. Faith answered. And lo, no one was there."

I hope you are excited. The adventure is just beginning! We pray that throughout this book, whenever you feel the unction, you will let out a holy roar! I will close with this paragraph from our book *Rebuilding the Altar*.

> Your voice matters now more than ever. Will you speak up? Dare we say to our kids that our nation was destroyed because we who called ourselves believers in Jesus were not willing to pay the price for speaking up? Will they look back and declare that we were loud for the wrong reasons and cowered in the harvest season? We must speak up before we miss our moment. Let history declare that we were those who chose holiness over heathenism and purpose over procrastination. This is our now! We must rise up and lead a Holy Spirit revolution.[5]

Rise up, lions!

CHAPTER 2

DO YOU TRUST ME?

Some trust in chariots and some in horses, but
we trust in the name of the LORD our God.
—PSALM 20:7

WHEN WAS THE last time you asked yourself, Whom or what do I trust? God desires that we trust Him. Yet many of us unwittingly live with very little trust in God in the midst of fear. Fear is most often based on our perception of what may happen rather than what is actually happening. For instance, we may fear for our future when we have no trust in our financial situation, or fear for our marriage when trust has been lost. We fear failure when we have not succeeded in past situations or when we feel ill-equipped. We fear embarrassment when we are not fully prepared to step up and lead. We tend to fear sickness or death or possible accidents. Oftentimes our human nature is to fear what others think about us or how we are viewed in other people's eyes. Fear is a powerful emotion that exerts significant influence over behavior, decisions, mental health, and relationships with others. When fear is in charge, we begin to live life looking over our shoulders, expecting the worst instead of the best.

To move from a life of fear to one of faith and trust in God, we first need to understand that God is absolutely trustworthy. Those who put their trust in Him can live lives of freedom, boldness, courage, and proper influence. So how does one move from fear to faith? It begins with a decision to live courageously. I have heard it said, "Fear is a reaction. Courage is a decision."[1] Courage comes when you have something or someone you can fully trust. The problem is that most of us only trust ourselves, and we all know how well that works out!

There is only one we can put all our trust, our hope, and our confidence in, and that is God alone. The prophet Jeremiah proclaimed, "But blessed is the one who trusts in the Lord, whose confidence is in him. They will be like a tree planted by the water that sends out its roots by the stream. It does not fear when heat comes; its leaves are always green. It has no worries in a year of drought and never fails to bear fruit" (Jer. 17:7–8). God is faithful and trustworthy, a never-ending stream that gives life to all who trust in Him. Sometimes the journey to that place of trust is a difficult one because the enemy wants to keep us living in a place of fear.

As I (Karen) stood at the kitchen sink one evening doing dishes after our family meal, I heard the words, "Do you trust Me?" That question was quickly followed by more as the Spirit of God spoke to me, saying, "You are about to walk through a difficult and uncertain season, Karen." I would love to say I quickly turned my ear toward heaven and listened intently. The truth of the matter is that I immediately rebuked those words as if it were the enemy who spoke them to me. Once again God spoke and said, "Karen, you are about to enter into a difficult and uncertain season, but do you trust Me?" In that moment, I knew it was the Spirit of God. Overwhelmed, I didn't know what to think. What could possibly be coming around the corner that would be difficult and uncertain in my life? I had faced other difficult situations and overcome other obstacles before. Yet this felt different. All of a sudden fear tried to enter my life and get me to imagine all sorts of devastating scenarios. My blood pressure rose, and my heart began to beat faster.

I must confess I have struggled with trust throughout my life, and like many with trust issues I tend to find it difficult to ask for help. My reaction to life's difficulties is often to try to figure out everything on my own and deal with it in my own strength. This generally causes frustration because it takes so much longer to handle the difficulty than if I had just trusted God with it in the first place. As I stood there at the sink wrestling with what I was hearing from God, my trust issues kicked in big-time. In that moment, God lovingly spoke again. "Do you trust Me, Karen? Do you trust who I am? Do you trust that I can get you from point A to point Z? Do you trust that I have already been where you are about to go and have already paved a safe path for you?"

As God's words began to register in my heart and mind, it became clear that God's focus was not on the actual challenge that lay ahead so much as the issue of trust. Was I willing to trust God? That was the question that sent me on a journey to address the fear and trust issues that had haunted me for decades. I was going to find out what trusting God really looked like, but it meant I would need the courage to take the first step. After all, fear is the nemesis of trust. As I pondered God's question to me, I wondered why He didn't ask me about my faith. Why was the question about trust? Throughout my life I've always considered faith and trust to be pretty much the same thing. However, this season in life was about to give me quite the lesson in the difference between faith and trust. Our family was about to enter a season that would test our faith and our trust in God, and He figured I needed to know the difference!

TRUSTING GOD

When he had been captured by his enemies, David wrote, "When I am afraid, I put my trust in you" (Ps. 56:3). Maybe you are reading this and you realize you have a bit of an issue with the topic of trust too. Trust can be difficult. Have you ever confused faith and trust or considered them the same thing? Perhaps someone has hurt you or betrayed your trust. Perhaps the events of your life have caused you to take matters into your own hands because you don't trust anyone with your future. We tend to base trust off past experiences or painful events in our lives.

I want to take a moment to clarify the differences between faith and trust. They are very similar and yet distinctly different. It is important to understand the difference in order to understand the need for both. *Merriam-Webster* defines *faith* as "allegiance to duty or a person"; "belief and trust in and loyalty to God"; and "firm belief in something for which there is no proof."[2] Faith is a spiritual decision based on a belief in something or someone without seeing it or having any tangible proof of its validity. You believe it because you know in your heart and your spirit that it is in fact the truth. The Bible says this about faith in Hebrews 11:1: "Now faith is the substance of things hoped for, the evidence of things not seen" (NKJV). Faith means I know that I know that I know God is real. I know God is with me. I know God can heal, deliver, and set me free. I cannot see Him with my physical eyesight, but my belief goes beyond human comprehension. My faith is a result of my encounter with God because something changed in me when I encountered God that caused me to never doubt Him.

Trust goes a little bit further. It is different in that trust requires something more, something deeper. Trust requires relationship. Trust is complete reliance and confidence in the integrity, strength, and ability of something or someone based on personal experience. To trust is "to hope or expect confidently" or to go somewhere or to do something without fear of consequences.[3] Trust is one of the most precious things in this world. It can take years to earn and be lost in a moment. We tend to trust people who are good to us, who have integrity, and whose actions line up with what they say.

Trust is all about relationship. While faith is believing without seeing, trust is knowing based on personal experience. Take marriage for example. When two people get married, they have faith that their spouse will be faithful and prioritize the marriage. As we know, all too often that trust gets broken. At the time of this writing, Pat and I have been married for twenty-nine years. During that time, we have developed a level of trust I never thought possible. Around every corner, in every situation and circumstance, it has been proven over and over that we will love each other, cherish each other, be there for each other, be faithful to each other, and laugh and enjoy the journey together. Our trust has grown to a point where we can rely on each other and have full confidence in one another. We are truly best friends. I could not imagine facing life without him, and I can face anything with him by my side. Our personal experience has built a strong foundation of trust.

Up until the encounter at the kitchen sink I thought I knew about trust. That was why it surprised me when God challenged my trust in Him. Of course He knows me much better than I know myself. His response to my why was simple: "Karen," He said, "you tend to rely on your own ability to fix things when you are afraid. I'm asking you to fully rely on Me, to have confidence in My plan and My character and My integrity and My process, without interfering or trying to fix things yourself. I want you to learn to act from a place of trust, not out of fear of the outcome. I'm asking you to draw from your personal experience and relationship with Me in order to trust Me because I have never failed you. Will you trust Me?"

God was calling me into a deeper relationship with Him, a place where I could stand unshaken by the storms of life, not because of my own ability but because of who He is. I was about to learn that peace resides at the intersection of faith and trust. Before it was all over, fear would have to take a back seat to make room for peace. As Isaiah 26:3 says, "You will keep in perfect peace those whose minds are steadfast, because they trust in you." Peace cannot be found in reliance on yourself, a job, doctors, positions, or titles. It is not found in being able to control your circumstances or having all the answers. Peace can only be found in total surrender and trust in God, in total reliance on the only One who does have all the answers. Faith is critical. It is the embryo of trust, the beginning that leads us into relationship with the only One who is totally trustworthy. With faith we can make the journey to trust.

God was asking me a serious question that evening at the kitchen sink. To jump-start the process of finding the answer, He directed me to pull out my mental photo album and take a walk down memory lane with Him, to remember how trustworthy He had been in my life. I was about to face the unknown in the form of a very difficult and uncertain situation, and God knew I would need more than faith. I was going to need complete and absolute trust in Him to get to the other side. He was asking me to turn the pages of life with Him and look at the memory of the two of us over the years. It started on a bench in the school courtyard. I was thirteen years old and needed to hear Him tell me I was not alone. I remember God saying, "I will never leave you, Karen." I wrote about the park bench encounter in *Dehydrated*. God wanted me to remember He knew my name, He saw my need, and my life mattered to Him.

Then He took me to a scene in our car so I could remember once again how He was with me just moments before I had a head-on collision. Our two-year-old son, Nate, was in the car with me that day. Moments before the crash I asked God to let Nate know how much He loved him and that He was real, and God did! Minutes before impact, from his car seat Nate said, "Mommy, Jesus just gave me a kiss and a hug." We should have died that day, but God preserved our lives. Nate is now leading a powerful youth movement in Modesto, California, at The House Modesto, led by Pastor Glen Berteau.

As I stood there with God, more memories flooded my heart, overwhelming me with God's goodness. There was our longed-for second child, Abby, who came to us from China after we spent eight years praying for God to give us a child. God gave me a vision of our daughter, waiting on us to come get her in China to make our home complete. I remembered the moment when Abby ran into the living room at five years old and told me Jesus visited her in a dream. He reminded her He also came to her when she was in the orphanage, telling her He was sending her forever mommy and daddy to come get her. Now our beautiful gift Abby has turned into a beautiful young woman who loves God passionately. God reminded me of our son, Nate, having spinal reconstructive surgery almost five years ago. I heard His voice that day as fear tried to overtake me. God said to me, "I am the same God today in the operating room as I was in the back seat of the car when Nate was two years old."

Suddenly it hit me: my loving Father God wasn't insulting me by asking if I trusted Him. He was asking me to take a walk down memory lane with Him to remind me of our relationship, to remind me of His character and unfailing love and how He has never once abandoned me or failed me. He reminded me of Psalm 9:10: "Those who know your name trust in you, for you, O LORD, do not abandon those who search for you" (NLT). He was reminding me that I know Him, that He is not an idea or a concept or an idol or a token. He is the real, living, breathing, all-powerful, all-knowing God. I know Him, and He knows me. Sometimes that is all we need.

That day at the sink God did not ask me, "Do you have faith, Karen?" Our relationship was past that point. He knew I believed in Him. He was asking me to pull from something deeper and more intimate, to go forward with total confidence and reliance on Him—and to do it without fear, based on the knowledge that He had been with me my whole life and never once failed me. I had seen Him move mountains before, so why should I doubt Him going forward? God was asking me to not focus on the storm, to keep my eyes on Him, and to trust Him to get me to the place of safety.

Jesus has already paved the path to safety in the darkness. There is nowhere we can go where He has not already been. Our own strength, abilities, gifts, talents, wisdom, and intellect cannot get us where we need to go during the times we cannot see the light for the darkness. Courage is often birthed in the darkness. If we will keep our eyes on the One who knows the way, we will always reach safety. Our strength in these seasons will come from God alone.

As God and I walked down memory lane, I knew we had the history between us to warrant my full trust. Isaiah 40:31 says this so well: "But those who trust in the LORD will find new strength. They will soar high on wings like eagles. They will run and not grow weary. They will walk and not faint" (NLT). Over the next year and a half, when I found myself getting weary and tired and wanting to give up, I would remember this moment and this scripture. It would remind me that trusting God is where true strength comes from. Our moments in private with God are where our strength in trials comes from. Our strength in public is birthed from secret encounters in the dark times.

FEAR COMES KNOCKING

Upon the leading of the Holy Spirit, we moved our family and our ministry from Birmingham, Alabama, to Fort Worth, Texas, in August 2017 to make it easier for us to travel. Once we arrived and settled in, I (Karen) began to develop some physical symptoms that I could not explain. These symptoms quickly began to interfere with daily life. I developed a continuous cough that made it difficult to speak at times. My joints, muscles, and bones began to ache. I began to get headaches, and I felt run-down and lacked energy on most days. To be honest, I dismissed most of these symptoms as mere exhaustion. We had moved to another state and recently launched our book *Rebuilding the Altar*. In the midst of all of these changes we were continuing to travel weekly, speaking at conferences and conventions and doing interviews for the new book. Who wouldn't be a bit run-down, right?

Eventually it became obvious I should get checked out by a doctor. I made an appointment and had some blood work done. After reviewing my symptoms, the doctor was a little concerned that there might be an underlying issue going on. He wanted to send me to a rheumatologist to check for several autoimmune disorders, including lupus, and Lyme disease. I was not too concerned at that point. I thought I was probably just a little vitamin deficient and needed more rest. The rheumatologist confirmed I did not have lupus or Lyme disease. All of my tests came back normal, except one. There was one test that looked suspicious, indicating an issue with my blood. When I asked what that meant, the doctor simply replied, "I am referring you to a hematologist-oncologist for further testing." No one wants to hear the word *oncologist*.

It is incredibly easy to talk about having faith when you are not the one in the middle of the crisis. It is so easy to throw out scriptures on faith and trust when you are not the one desperately needing to put into practice what you claim to believe. My next visit to the doctor drastically challenged the level of faith I previously walked in. Have you ever sat quietly, wondering if you have been a fraud in your faith because all of a sudden a whole new level of faith is being required of you? Have you ever had to dig into the depths of your spirit to revive and reignite the flame of faith because you were dealt a blow you did not see coming, the breath has been knocked out of you, and you feel lost and disoriented in the moment? That is how I felt when the oncologist came in and told me my blood had too many red blood cells and that it showed one of the rarest mutated genes present in leukemia. *Leukemia!*

Fear took center stage. Did you know that fear loves an audience? And when it gets one, it will have you thinking of every possible horrible scenario. I had to dig deep to pull faith and trust up out of the darkness trying to swallow us. Pat and I decided on that very first visit to reject the cancer diagnosis. By that I mean we refused to name it or take any kind of ownership of it. It is like having one of your kids bring home a stray dog. Everyone knows that if you name it, you will keep it! We did not plan on keeping this diagnosis. It was a lie from the enemy and a distraction from our destiny. The Bible tells us in John 8:44 that the devil is a liar: "He was a murderer from the beginning, not holding to the truth, for there is no truth in him. When he lies, he speaks his native language, for he is a liar and the father of lies." As children of God we must stop accepting everything the enemy sends our way as absolute truth. We must develop a "not today, devil" mentality that breaks the cycle of panic and worry. We must create a new pattern of preparation before the storm.

From the very beginning we asked the doctor not to call my issue cancer or leukemia. Thankfully the doctor agreed to our request. The enemy hated the awakening that had taken place in our family and across the nation throughout the writing of our book *Rebuilding the Altar*. We faced challenges throughout the process of getting that book to print. Pat lost his voice and could barely talk for six weeks. Our daughter, Abby, began to have issues with her ears, and I had a disk rupture in my neck that required surgery. Now this. It was time to go to war and put into practice what we preached.

At the time, the doctor's plan of action was to monitor my blood and retest in a few weeks. When my blood was retested, it showed the same issue and the same rare mutated gene. Doctor's visit after doctor's visit the issue with my blood and the rare mutated cancer gene remained. Trust did not mean we lived in denial but rather that we understood the final say belonged to God. My symptoms continued, but something began to arise in our family. A boldness and a courage were awakened from deep within our spirits. My forty-ninth birthday was just around the corner, and Pat kept asking me what gift I wanted. I truly could not think of anything I wanted or needed until a week before my birthday. After my prayer time one morning I felt the Holy Spirit ask me, "Are you tired of being afraid? Are you ready to fight back?" It was as if a light bulb went on, and suddenly I knew the one gift I wanted more than anything. With a cancer diagnosis hanging over my head, there was one thing I wanted to do on my birthday—to kick the devil in the face! So that is exactly what we did.

LEARNING TO BE OVERCOMERS

God spoke to me about starting a biweekly Facebook Live program with one purpose: to walk out what we knew to be true—that in Christ we are victorious overcomers. We were not to sulk or even tell anyone about the cancer. Every episode would focus on defeating fear and the lies of the enemy. Whoever tuned in would be invited to walk with us as we learned to be overcomers. We wanted others to understand we do not have to be victims. We are more than conquerors through Christ Jesus who loves us (Rom. 8:37). By walking together, we could keep one another accountable on the journey.

It is hard to give up when people are watching you

and are on the journey with you. As I focused on helping others, I became less absorbed by my own issue. Suddenly the victory was for more than just me. The battle would be won for everyone stuck in the middle of fear. When one wins, we all win. Fear is simply a ploy of the enemy to distract us from our purpose. When we defeat fear, we defeat the enemy. We are all looking for peace and something to hope for or trust in during times of anxiety. If the future feels uncertain right now, and fear, worry, and anxiety seem to be taking up too much room in your heart and mind, know this: God is already in all of your tomorrows, waiting on you to get there. You can walk in full reliance and confidence because He knows the way and has already mapped out the course for victory.

If you find it difficult to trust God, then it is time to get to know Him better, to press in to a deeper relationship with Him. Invite Him into your life and start a memory album. Allow Him to show you who He is and who you are in Him. God wants to walk with you on this great adventure called life and teach you to embrace every part of the journey. He will never ask you to figure it out on your own. There is power in trusting Him that brings clarity and light through the dark times. God sees around the other side of the mountain where we cannot fully see. He promises to make our paths straight (Prov. 3:6). The journey can either make you bitter and fearful, or it can build courage and strength. It all depends on whom you trust. No matter what form fear has taken in your life, you were created to overcome. David, a man well familiar with the heat of battle, wrote:

Let the morning bring me word of your unfailing love, for I have put my trust in you. Show me the way I should go, for to you I entrust my life.
—PSALM 143:8

Make a decision today to choose to trust God, for He has never lost a battle. He has never failed. God will never leave you or forsake you. His Word is always true. He "is not a man, that He should lie" (Num. 23:19, NKJV). We can believe Him when He says, "And be sure of this; I am with you always, even to the end of the age" (Matt. 28:20, NLT). Don't focus on the issue or the battle. Instead confront the liar, remembering that fear is the thief of trust. Trust begins with relationship. When you truly trust God, you will see miraculous signs and wonders. God is waiting to break the cycle of fear not only for you but your family for generations to come. Your freedom will teach the next generation how to trust God.

CHAPTER 3

THE FORMULA FOR DEFEATING FEAR

God has not given us a spirit of fear, but of power and of love and of a sound mind.

—2 Timothy 1:7, NKJV

O UR RELATIONSHIP WITH God should always be one of continual growth and reaching new levels of faith and understanding. As we learn to trust God, it becomes easier to take Him at His word. I (Karen) am a firm believer that God works everything for our good. The Bible declares this to be true: "And we know that in all things God works for the good of those who love him, who have been called according to his purpose" (Rom. 8:28). I have adopted this scripture as a motto in my life. As you press in to the issue of trusting God and come into a fuller understanding of fear and how it can be used to turn the tables on the enemy, I believe you will come to the realization, just as I did, that as believers we don't have to settle for anything less than the fullness of what God has for us.

If the devil throws lemons in your life, please do not

make lemonade. Throw the lemons back in the devil's face and demand an espresso, as expressed in John 10:10: "The thief's purpose is to steal and kill and destroy. My purpose is to give them a rich and satisfying life" (NLT). God never asks you to settle for lemonade. He wants to give you the full-on espresso life experience. This is the reason Pat and I rejected the cancer diagnosis. Cancer was not part of a full, rich, and satisfying life. Therefore, we threw it back in the devil's face!

After the initial diagnosis of my condition I continued to have blood tests over the next couple of months, but there was no change. Doubt wanted to creep in when we didn't see the results we were looking for. There were days when we had to spend more time praying and reading the Word of God to keep our minds from giving in to the fear that wanted to overtake us. When doubts tried to flood in, we ran straight into the presence of God for shelter. It was there, in the peace and quiet of the shadow of His presence, that all other shadows faded and we were able to hear God's voice. Psalm 91:1–2 says, "Those who live in the shelter of the Most High will find rest in the shadow of the Almighty. This I declare about the LORD: He alone is my refuge, my place of safety; he is my God, and I trust him" (NLT).

This beautiful promise and firm declaration gave us great strength. When you learn to run into and reside in the shelter of the Most High God, you begin to realize that the darkness around you might just be the shadow of His wings. During this season, God began to show me simple yet amazing truths that set me free from the grip of fear. As I was able to hear His voice more clearly, the voice of the enemy grew weaker. You see, fear is nothing more than a straw man set before us by the enemy, a learned or perceived aberration that can grow into an absolute if we allow it to. God wanted me to understand that fear is not the absence of courage. In fact fear is the embryo of courage! Fear is courage waiting to be awakened.

Without the presence of fear we have no need for courage. Without a real enemy we have no need for courage to be awakened. Within the child of God who is full of faith, there is a roar waiting to be released. If you will listen, God will lead you into a place of intimacy with Him that will change your walk with Him and awaken the roar in you. Perhaps you are blaming God today for your circumstances, or your issues have caused you to shrink back in fear. Maybe fear has so gripped you that you are flailing in a sea of panic and even hysteria, not knowing which way to turn. When our confidence and security have been snatched from us, our first reaction can be to hide in the dark. Fear and isolation can lead us straight into the enemy's grip. Yet God says we are to fear not.

"Do not be afraid" is one of the most repeated commands in the Bible. That tells me God never intended for us to go even a day with fear as our companion. He wants to be our daily companion; He does not want us to walk in fear. That is why He says, "Fear not, for I am with you; be not dismayed, for I am your God. I will strengthen you, yes, I will help you, I will uphold you with My righteous right hand" (Isa. 41:10, NKJV).

How does God strengthen us? How does He uphold us with His mighty right hand? He does it through His Word and His Spirit. Just read 2 Timothy 1:7: "God has not given us a spirit of fear, but of power and of love and of a sound mind" (NKJV). Honestly I don't know how many times I have read that scripture and failed to grasp its full meaning. Then one morning during my devotional time, as I encountered this scripture yet again, I felt the gentle nudging of the Spirit to pause and camp out on those words. As I did, something struck me differently. In the past I tended to grab hold of the first part of the verse but not the second. I was rejecting the spirit of fear but not allowing God to replace it with His power and love that leads to a sound mind.

When we just fulfill a spiritual obligation by reading God's Word instead of waiting for His presence to enliven the words in our hearts and minds, we miss much of what God has for us. Everything we need for living, including knowledge and strategy for the battle, is in His Word. I didn't know it at the time, but 2 Timothy 1:7 would become a key scripture in my life.

A SUPERNATURAL LIFESTYLE

I will never forget. It was near the turning of the year from 2017 to 2018, and Pat and I were just driving and dreaming together. As we drove, Pastor John Kilpatrick called with a prophetic word for us. He spoke incredible truth to us that day, but one statement in particular stood out to me. It was really a question, and since that day, I have pondered and referred back to it often. He said, "Why are Christians always looking to the natural and the obvious for answers when God always works in the supernatural?"

Good question! Don't we always look to the natural first? Then, after exhausting our natural resources, we finally turn to God. If we are not attentive to God, we may miss things He wants to reveal to us beyond our natural comprehension. If we would only trust in His ways and not our own, we would gain the supernatural strength and courage needed for the journey. He specifically says in Isaiah 55:8–9: "My thoughts are nothing like your thoughts....And my ways are far beyond anything you could imagine. For just as the heavens are higher than the earth, so my ways are higher than your ways and my thoughts higher than your thoughts" (NLT).

Because God's ways are so far beyond our imagination, we have no choice but to believe beyond what we perceive in the natural. Yet, although His thoughts and ways are beyond our imagination, we need only ask and He will give us wisdom and understanding. God will open the windows of heaven for you if you will simply ask and then listen and receive. "If any of you lacks wisdom, you should ask God, who gives generously to all without finding fault, and it will be given to you" (Jas. 1:5). You see, the Word of God is living and active. It is the very breath of God and all-powerful. The writer of Hebrews declared, "For the word of God is quick, and powerful, and sharper than any twoedged sword, piercing even to the dividing asunder of soul and spirit, and of the joints and marrow, and is a discerner of the thoughts and intents of the heart" (Heb. 4:12, KJV).

With that knowledge 2 Timothy 1:7 can be seen in a whole new light. Let's begin with the first part of verse 7. First and foremost, God did not give us a spirit of fear.

Fear comes from our adversary, the devil. Second, God did give us something *instead* of fear because He knew the enemy was sculpting fear as a weapon to take us out. If the enemy is going to forge a weapon, you can believe God has forged something more powerful to defeat the enemy. Because God is all-knowing and all-powerful, He sees the feeble attempts of the enemy and already has our escape strategy in place. He does not leave us helpless or ill-equipped for the battle. Here are His words from Isaiah 54:17: "'No weapon forged to be used against you will succeed; you will refute everyone who tries to accuse you. This is what the LORD will do for his servants—I will vindicate them,' says the LORD" (NET). *The Message* paraphrases that scripture to say, "No weapon that can hurt you has *ever* been forged" (emphasis added). This is what we need to know from 2 Timothy 1:7—that the enemy does indeed forge weapons, but none of them will be successful in taking us out.

WEAPONS OF OUR WARFARE

Let's look a little further at the second part of verse 7 in 2 Timothy 1. Not only did God not give us a spirit of fear, He actually gave us an arsenal of weapons to defeat fear. God provided not just one but three distinct weapons that enable us to combat, conquer, overtake, and destroy fear. The Bible tells us exactly what those weapons are. Instead of fear God gives us power, love, and a sound mind. Each of these three possesses a specific ability to bring us back into a relationship of trust with God the Father, enabling us then to focus on His power, His character, and His ways. When we utilize power, love, and a sound mind in the face of fear, it reminds us of our relationship standing with the Father. When we wield God's weapons, the enemy no longer sees us but rather God in us.

Fear will try to greet you every morning and work toward creating an absolute in your life. With cancer looming in the shadows of my life, I needed to know what weapons had been given to me to fight this war. I needed to know I was not left vulnerable to the enemy's schemes. I needed to understand that fear was not meant to be my companion. I had to kick fear to the curb or it would kick me to the curb! Together Pat and I rejected every bad report from the doctor. We would bring the report home and lay it on the wooden altar in our bedroom. Every negative diagnosis and every negative report was laid on the altar along with our prayers. Just as King David did, together we would declare: "Every morning you'll hear me at it again. Every morning I lay out the pieces of my life on your altar and watch for fire to descend" (Ps. 5:3, MSG).

The enemy's fear will leave you broken and fragmented. But God's fire will take what is broken and weld it back together again. If the enemy is trying to break you to pieces and leave you desperate for deliverance, healing, hope, and freedom in your mind, lay the pieces of your life on the altar today and let the fire of God's glory come down and burn up what does not belong and what is not meant for you. Then let what remains come out as pure gold. God has placed His weapons of warfare in your hands. Use them and know that your enemy is a defeated foe! Let's look at each of these weapons individually to understand them more fully.

Power

The word for *power* in the Greek is *dunamis*.[1] It is the word from which we get the term *dynamite*.[2] This connection demonstrates what God wants to be obvious and intentional—we have a weapon that can blow up the plans of the enemy. *Dunamis* also refers to the ability to do powerful deeds, miracles, and marvelous works.[3] The word *power* itself means the "ability to direct or influence the behavior of others or the course of events."[4] In other words, we have the power to change the atmosphere! The enemy must capitulate in the presence of God!

Love

At first glance love can seem like an unlikely weapon. Yet it actually is one of the most powerful weapons of all. Let's consider 1 John 4:18 to see how specific God is when describing love and what it does. "There is no fear in love. But perfect love drives out fear." Notice that the scripture says "perfect" love. God is the only one whose love is perfect. We can look at 1 John 4:8 to understand this better. It states, "Whoever does not love does not know God, because God is love." It follows that if we know God, then we have His perfect love in us. If we look further in 1 John 4:15–16, it becomes even clearer: "If anyone acknowledges that Jesus is the Son of God, God lives in them and they in God. And so we know and rely on [trust] the love God has for us. God is love. Whoever lives in love lives in God, and God in them."

John is saying here that love is based on relationship and trust. This passage in 1 John is pointing us back to the very origin of love. God *is* love. Did you catch that? Perfect love is a part of and comes from the most beautiful, most valuable, most satisfying, most powerful being that exists—God. That is a pretty powerful weapon, don't you think?

Let's look quickly at another aspect of what the Bible says about love. Did you know that Scripture actually gives a definition for love in 1 Corinthians 13:4–7?

> Love is patient, love is kind. It does not envy, it does not boast, it is not proud. It does not dishonor others, it is not self-seeking, it is not easily angered, it keeps no record of wrongs. Love does not delight in evil but rejoices with the truth. It always protects, always trusts, always hopes, always perseveres.

I cannot recall another word so vividly described in Scripture. Evidently it is an important concept for us to comprehend.

Sound mind

Our third weapon is a sound mind. As I dug deep into God's intention for this weapon, I began to gain understanding that transformed my thought process and profoundly affected how I approached my cancer diagnosis. I learned to rely on God instead of trusting in my own strength. God wanted me to take authority over what

I allowed to enter my thoughts and what I allowed to be spoken over me. When we walk in fear, no matter the reason, we tend to think irrationally at times. We tend to think there must be something wrong with us, and we grasp quickly for anything to relieve our anxiety. If we continue down that path, we will soon feel out of control. When that happens, we make decisions from a place of panic and from a survival mentality rather than trusting God. For this very reason it is important to understand the weapon of having a sound mind as described in 2 Timothy 1:7.

The concept of a sound mind in this context comes from the Greek word *sōphrōn*, which is a compound of the words *sōzō* and *phrēn*.[5] *Sōzō* is Greek for *save* and means to deliver, protect, and keep sound.[6] *Phrēn* means understanding and is sometimes translated "mind."[7] These two words taken together, as in 2 Timothy 1:7, mean "sound mind." The idea presented by *sōphrōn* is that a mind that is saved and protected is a sound mind, one that has been delivered, rescued, revived, salvaged, protected, and brought into a place of safety and security so that it is no longer affected by illogical, unfounded, and absurd thoughts, a mind that is thinking correctly.[8] Because God has given us a sound mind, we can think correctly about how to live in these last days.

Based on this information regarding power, love, and a sound mind, let us look again at 2 Timothy 1:7:

> God has not given us a spirit of fear [panic], but of power [the ability to see miraculous signs and wonders and the ability to direct and influence the course of events to change the atmosphere] and of

love [to cast out fear by waiting patiently on God's promises because I am fully protected, as I always trust, always hope, and always persevere!] and of a sound mind [that is delivered, rescued, revived, salvaged, protected, and brought into a place of safety and security so that it is no longer affected by illogical, unfounded, and absurd thoughts].

This is why we can boldly declare 2 Corinthians 10:5—that we are "casting down imaginations and every high thing that exalts itself against the knowledge of God, bringing every thought into captivity to the obedience of Christ" (MEV).

I pray this is starting to come together for you now. Can you see how these weapons are given to us so we will be fully equipped to withstand any attack the enemy brings our way? Throughout the Scriptures, God remains consistent in His character. In relationship with Him we can fully rely on what He says and know that it is true. God's Word has been proven throughout history. He has never bounced a check. We can stand on His Word and take it to the bank just like it says in Numbers 23:19: "God is not a man, so he does not lie. He is not human, so he does not change his mind. Has he ever spoken and failed to act? Has he ever promised and not carried it through?" (NLT).

The revelation about 2 Timothy 1:7 brought life to me as I walked through one of the scariest times of my life. Pat had it printed onto two posters, one for his office and one for mine. Every day I read it and declared it over my life. It became my fight song! With God's weapons of power, love, and a sound mind, we can cast down every imagination (aberration) and every high thing that exalts itself against the knowledge of God. The cancer coming against my body was just that—an aberration conjured up by Satan himself. And we refused to give in to fear.

CHAPTER 4

WHEN THE SHADOW LOOMS

Whatever is good and perfect is a gift coming down to us from God our Father, who created all the lights in the heavens. He never changes or casts a shifting shadow.

—JAMES 1:17, NLT

THE MOMENT WE dreaded had finally come. The doctor let us know he would no longer wait to take a bone marrow biopsy. He was so compassionate and had agreed to put it off each time I (Karen) asked because I was believing for my healing. I didn't want the findings of the biopsy to cause my faith to waver. I was scheduled to fly overseas to speak at the Herdeira conference with Pastors Marco and Juçara Peixoto of CEIZS church in Brazil, and I absolutely did not want to have a bone marrow biopsy before I left. We agreed that I would have the procedure a few days after I returned from Brazil. Shortly before the Brazil trip, we took a week of rest at the beach. The beach is our happy place, and we came home refreshed by the Lord. When I left for Brazil, I was stirred in my spirit for all that God was going to do in that beautiful country.

I had spoken at the Herdeira conference once before and absolutely fell in love with the beautiful, fierce, brilliant women and their passion for God's presence. As the first morning of the conference approached, I found myself questioning the message I was set to preach about the woman with the issue of blood from Mark 5. I wanted to point out that she not only had faith and trust in God for her healing, but she also actually became a catalyst for revival as her faith awakened faith in those who witnessed her healing. I was planning to preach about what was going on in my life, even though I had not yet seen my healing manifest.

That morning, the enemy began to mock and taunt me, attacking my confidence and authenticity. I pushed through, and as my name was called and I began to walk up to the platform, the enemy whispered in my ear, "You're a fraud. You're a fake. You are preaching a lie. *You have cancer!*" I knew these thoughts were completely unfounded. Yet I froze in my steps for a moment, taken aback by what I was hearing.

Then suddenly a holy anger and boldness rose up in me. I began to quote 2 Timothy 1:7 and declare power, love, and a sound mind to be active in my life. I declared the enemy a liar and that I was changing the atmosphere for the supernatural to take place. I told the enemy I was protected and would continue to hope, trust, and persevere. I told the enemy, "No! I am walking out the Word of God. I am the woman with the issue of blood who is deciding today to leave her prison of fear to run after the trusted truth of who God is. In Him I live and move and have my being [Acts 17:28]. Today, I am revival, and all those here will be witnesses to who God is."

I reached the platform, walked over to the podium, and opened my notes. The moment I opened my notes, the same loving voice that spoke to me at the kitchen sink the previous year spoke to me again. The Spirit of God said, "Karen, today your blood has been healed." At the exact same time, in Charlotte, North Carolina, where Pat was preaching, God spoke to him as well, saying, "Pat, the storm is over." I flew home from Brazil, and Pat and Abby flew home from where Pat had been ministering that weekend. We were prepared for the bone marrow biopsy that awaited me the day after we returned, knowing our perfect Father in heaven was in complete control. We knew that "whatever is good and perfect is a gift coming down to us from God our Father, who created all the lights in the heavens. He never changes or casts a shifting shadow" (Jas. 1:17, NLT).

THE PARALYSIS OF ANALYSIS

Have you ever said to yourself, "I feel like something bad is going to happen"? These feelings are the shadows, the what-ifs. They have the power to paralyze us into believing we are not safe, or our future is at risk, or our loved ones are in danger. I (Pat) call it the paralysis of analysis. These looming shadows of dread and doubt become faint whispers that haunt the soul and bring fear. And as you know, fear is one of the main weapons the enemy uses to keep us in the dark. Once this battle of the mind sets itself up, it has the power to cage your spirit behind the steel bars of doubt, insecurity, and fear. Remember, *fear is a learned or perceived aberration that grows into an absolute.*

The Bible tells us we have the power to cast down these attacks: "For though we walk in the flesh, we do not war according to the flesh. For the weapons of our warfare are not carnal but mighty in God for pulling down strongholds, casting down arguments and every high thing that exalts itself against the knowledge of God, bringing every thought into captivity to the obedience of Christ" (2 Cor. 10:3–5, NKJV). In other words, the Bible is telling us we have the power to open the back door in our brains and shove out the lies of the enemy.

That is exactly what God was telling Karen when He asked her to trust Him during her toughest season. He was teaching both of us to discipline our minds to dismiss the lies of the enemy. God knows that over time our perceptions (the whispers of the enemy) can become more real than what is really taking place in our reality. As long as we listen to the lies of the enemy, we won't step into the destiny God has for us.

Faith is the antidote to fear. It is our blindness, our inability to see what is next, that God uses to teach us to declare, "I trust You, God!" as we fall on our knees in prayer, lifting our hands in honor and surrendering our hearts with abandon to the only One who is worthy. God is calling us to "live by faith, not by sight" (2 Cor. 5:7). When we do, we start living under the shadow of the Almighty, not in the shadowland of the enemy. Let me share with you three ways I have learned to defeat the shadows of the enemy.

TURN ON THE LIGHT

"Daddy, there is something in my closet. I see a shadow. The shadow scares me." Those were the words I often heard coming from the room of our son, Nate, in the middle of the night when he was a young boy. I would get out of bed, barely awake, and make my way into his room to deal once again with the shadow monster. Each time this happened, I would find Nate, stricken with fear, huddled in his bed. The shadows of the night were trying to win the battle for his mind. I would turn on the light, sit on the side of the bed close to my trembling son, and pray. At times I sang to him. When this part of our routine was over, Nate would say, "Daddy, get the Holy Spirit spray."

I would then go over to the shelf in his room and grab the bottle of Holy Spirit spray. Karen and I had taken a water bottle and written "Holy Spirit Spray" on the side in black marker in an attempt to teach our son the power of the Holy Spirit over fear. You might be laughing to yourself as you read this, but don't knock it until you try it. Sleep deprivation can create innovation. I would then walk to the edge of the closet and begin to spray. With the appropriate amount of Holy Spirit spray released into the closet to deal with the shadow monster, I would end our routine with, "There you go, champ. The Holy Spirit just defeated whatever was trying to scare you." Nate would respond, "OK, Daddy. I love you." Then he would fall back to sleep.

Every one of us has access to a bottle of Holy Spirit spray. James 1:17 says, "Every good gift and every perfect gift is from above, and comes down from the Father of lights, with whom there is no variation or shadow of turning" (NKJV). When we are in need of the light, all we have to do is call upon the Father of lights. God is the One who gave birth to light. His shadow is the only shadow that matters. In Psalm 63 David said: "I lie awake each night thinking of you and reflecting on how you help me like a father. I sing through the night under your splendor-shadow, offering up to you my songs of delight and joy!" (vv. 6–7, TPT). God is calling us to the same childlike faith Nate had as a young boy. Jesus said in Matthew 18:3, "Unless you change and become like little children, you will never enter the kingdom of heaven." Why? Because children have an amazing ability to trust. A few squirts of Holy Spirit spray was all Nate needed to dispel the shadows. In Matthew 21:16 Jesus taught that the praise of a child is a weapon when He quoted Psalm 8:2: "Through the praise of children and infants you have established a stronghold against your enemies, to silence the foe and the avenger."

The fact of the matter is that true freedom comes when you make up your mind to live in the now! The psalmist said it best in Psalm 46:1–3 (TPT):

> God, you're such a safe and powerful place to find refuge! You're a proven help in time of trouble— more than enough and always available whenever I need you. So we will never fear even if every structure of support were to crumble away. We will not fear even when the earth quakes and

shakes, moving mountains and casting them into the sea. For the raging roar of stormy winds and crashing waves cannot erode our faith in you.

RESTORE YOUR PRAISE ROAD

Fear became a constant companion in my life at a very young age. As I (Pat) got older, I learned to mask it with humor, but it was always in the corner of my life. It really is a miracle that I have spoken on thousands of stages in front of crowds all over the world. In the early years of ministry travel there were times when I would be frozen with fear as I got ready to walk on stage to minister at large gatherings. I can actually remember walking behind the stage of large venues and calling Karen to ask her to pray over my nerves. That was until I found the weapon of praise!

Do you know that you can worship right past your fears? Worship became my nerve pill, replacing the thoughts of this world with the thoughts of God. In fact worship has become one of our family's greatest weapons against the schemes of the enemy. When you come into God's presence with worship, His joy will overtake you. Psalm 16:11 says, "You make known to me the path of life; in your presence there is fullness of joy; at your right hand are pleasures forevermore" (ESV).

When Karen was diagnosed with cancer, something awakened in me, sending me into battle mode with the enemy. I remember the day we got the news. We were very quiet on the way home from the doctor's office. Upon arriving back at the house, both of us began to make ourselves busy as we processed the diagnosis. I went from room to room, wandering aimlessly and shouting, "Satan, you're a liar!" Our old foe—fear—had arrived once again to try to wreak havoc upon our home. Yet something was different this time, as if an angel army had surrounded me. Instead of receding into discouragement, anger, and doubt, I heard the voice of God say, "Pat, we got this!" His words caused a spirit of resoluteness and war to arise from the core of my very being. "If it's a fight you want, Satan, then it's a fight you will get," I cried to the devil.

The enemy called fear was trying to overstep our destiny, and God awakened us to the battle! Every morning, as soon as I woke up, I turned on worship in the house, saying to the Echo Dots all over our house, "Alexa, play 'Surrounded' by Upper Room." Immediately the song would fill our house, giving us the courage we needed to face our day boldly. One of my favorite passages of Scripture is Psalm 62:1–6. I am quoting it here from the Passion Translation:

> I stand silently to listen for the one I love, waiting as long as it takes for the Lord to rescue me. For God alone has become my Savior. He alone is my safe place; his wrap-around presence always protects me. For he is my champion defender; there's no risk of failure with God. So why would I let worry paralyze me, even when troubles multiply around me? But look at these who want me dead, shouting their vicious threats at me! The moment they discover my weakness they all begin plotting to take me down. Liars, hypocrites, with nothing good to say. All of their energies are spent on

moving me from this exalted place. Pause in his presence

I am standing in absolute stillness, silent before the one I love, waiting as long as it takes for him to rescue me. Only God is my Savior, and he will not fail me. For he alone is my safe place. His wrap-around presence always protects me as my champion defender. There's no risk of failure with God!

In 2018 we took that week at the beach before we both flew off to minister, Karen to the Herdeira conference with Pastors Marco and Juçara Peixoto, and I to Pennsylvania and North Carolina. The beach is our happy place. We had been fighting this cancer battle but were growing weary and needed a rest. Weariness has a way of wearing out a person's will to fight. With the constant shadow of death (Ps. 23:4) over every aspect of our lives, "Surrounded (Fight My Battles)," the words of which are about defeating the enemy with worship, became our battle cry. The words pierced the shadows in our hearts, assuring us we were surrounded by God's love in the midst of our battle. God reminded us that although there was a war going on, victory was coming.

Even after Karen was healed, God continued to remind us that He is the source of our victory and that the battle belongs to the Lord. In early June we took another trip to the beach for a time of relaxation and celebration. One evening we heard music coming from outside on the beach. Curious, I opened the sliding glass door to investigate. The beach had been desolate all day, but there on the sand, six floors below our balcony, was a group of women worshipping. As they lifted their voices to heaven, a beautiful sound broke the quiet of the evening. They were singing "Surrounded (Fight My Battles)."

Sitting there on the balcony with the sweet and powerful strains of worship flooding our hearts, in that moment we knew God had sent those women to serenade us like a kiss from heaven. The very song we had listened to for months was now being sung right in front of our condo. The battle had been hard, but we had won by fighting on our knees. Karen posted a photo of this beautiful worship service on Instagram. We found out later that the group was from a church in Louisiana that was holding a women's retreat at the beach. Their pastor, Shane Warren from The Assembly in West Monroe, Louisiana, is a good friend of ours. How like our loving God to bring worship right to our doorstep—through a friend no less—as a sweet reminder of our victory in Him.

TAKE AUTHORITY OVER THE SHADOW

Ephesians 6:12 says, "For our struggle is not against flesh and blood, but against the rulers, against the authorities, against the powers of this dark world and against the spiritual forces of evil in the heavenly realms." Oftentimes we fail to recognize that what we are fighting in the natural is actually supernatural. Some shadows are not mirages but harassing demonic spirits sent from the enemy. God has given us the weapons we need to fight our battles. We must learn to open our spiritual eyes and see what the enemy is doing and what God is doing.

Jesus has given believers authority over demonic powers. "Behold, I give unto you power to tread on serpents and scorpions [Satan and demons], and over all the power of the enemy: nothing shall by any means hurt you. Notwithstanding in this rejoice not, that the spirits are subject unto you; but rather rejoice, because your names are written in heaven" (Luke 10:19–20, KJV). In Colossians 2:15 the apostle Paul tells us that Jesus Himself did this very thing: "And having disarmed the powers and authorities, he made a public spectacle of them, triumphing over them by the cross."

I will never forget the battle we faced in China when we adopted our daughter, Abby, and how it became an opportunity to exercise our God-given authority with victory. When we arrived in China, we were able at last to hold our daughter in our arms. However, the process of adoption wasn't complete, so we spent two weeks traveling to several provinces to complete the paperwork required for Abby to become ours. The first night at the hotel with our precious new daughter, our gift from heaven, was just magical. We couldn't believe God had trusted us with such a gift. Abby had several infections in her body, so we went to work to get her healthy.

During our second night as a family Abby began to experience what are known as night terrors. *Night terror* is defined as "a sleep disruption that seems similar to a nightmare, but is far more dramatic."[1] Abby began to wake up every couple of hours, screaming in fear. Every time she began to rest soundly again, a terror would hit her. This went on for several days, after which we were at our wits' end, not knowing what to do to help her. Exhausted and frazzled, we pushed on through the adoption process.

After days of no sleep I had had enough. We have this promise in Romans 16:20: "The God of peace will soon crush Satan under your feet. The grace of our Lord Jesus be with you" (NASB). Late one night, as the rest of the family slept, the Lord spoke to me, telling me to turn on some worship music on my laptop. I did so quietly, so as not to awaken anyone, and then I began to pray in the Spirit for my family. I was walking in James 4:7, which says, "Submit therefore to God. Resist the devil and he will flee from you" (NASB).

Suddenly I saw a giant demonic shadow standing in the corner of the hotel room. Instead of fear overtaking me, I experienced what I believe was righteous anger. The shadow was clearly evil. It was quite real, and it was tormenting my family. I pointed at the demonic figure and demanded it leave my daughter alone. "She now belongs to me, and my name is hers," I said. As I rebuked the demon and commanded it leave, I watched it go out the window of our hotel room. From that night on, our daughter has never experienced another night terror. As her father I exercised my God-given authority through Christ on her behalf.

The next day, as we traveled by plane to another province, Karen whispered to me, "I saw it."

"What are you talking about?" I asked.

"I saw the demon in the room," she said, "and I heard you command it to leave. I watched it go out the window and leave."

I was overcome with emotion as I realized I had an obligation and an authority to protect my family! I challenge you to take authority over your home and family. God has anointed you to walk in freedom and power. Stand firm and know that God will back you up. Tell Satan to get away from your house, your family, your marriage, your body, your finances, and your dreams. You are a temple, not a shack. God inhabits you. He has given you the authority to stop the enemy in his tracks. Don't delay! Take back your dominion! And never forget that the most dangerous Christian is the Christian who actually understands the weapons God has given us.

APPLY THE BLOOD OF JESUS

> For this purpose the Son of God was manifested,
> that He might destroy the works of the devil.
> —1 JOHN 3:8, NKJV

Growing up, every time my siblings and I left the house, my mother said, "I plead the blood of Jesus over you." She continues this practice even now that we are all grown well into adulthood. It is her declaration of protection from Revelation 12:11: "They triumphed over him by the blood of the Lamb and by the word of their testimony." Growing up I actually thought that all parents said this over their children until one of my friends heard her make this declaration and wanted to know what she was doing. "It's just my mom's way of dealing with worry about her children" was my reply. As I got older, I can honestly say there were times when that declaration caused me to change direction because I wanted to stay under the covering of God's protection.

Declaring the blood of Jesus was also how my mother defeated her personal deep fears that came from a life of pain. You see, our family story is pretty miraculous. It's definitely a "but for the grace of God" story. My parents received Christ when I was just a child and were radically delivered from a life of addiction and pain. They had grown up in Detroit, amidst the drug culture of the sixties and seventies. My father had been deeply involved in illegal activity and the mafia until Jesus saved him. Nevertheless, at a very young age and as young adults they experienced so much tragedy.

Did you know that tragedy has a trajectory? The painful memories from yesterday often determine whether we have peace today. As a result many believers live in fear that tomorrow will bring great pain or sorrow rather than trusting Jesus in the now. Jesus said in Matthew 6:34, "So don't worry about tomorrow, for tomorrow will bring its own worries. Today's trouble is enough for today" (NLT). I have often said that Jesus was crucified between two thieves who represented yesterday and tomorrow. There was Jesus in the midst of them, right smack in their "now."

We cannot change where we have been or what we have been through, but we can change how we let it control us. Our dear friend Dr. Wayne Scott Andersen once made a statement at a conference that stuck with me. He said, "Stop trying to have a better past." His words personally awakened me to the fact that so much of my past had control over my today. The same is true for many others who have built a monument of pain and sorrow at the place they were harmed or hurt the most. Instead of realizing we survived "the worst," we continually visit the tombstone of yesterday's pain, allowing its shadow to dictate the peace we walk in today. Far too often the greatest attacks against the spirit and mind come from the shadows that loom over life instead of the reality that God is still in charge.

It is impossible to look forward when you are busy fearing what is behind you. God wants you to look straight ahead. The apostle Paul said, "Forgetting the past and looking forward to what lies ahead, I press on to reach the end of the race and receive the heavenly prize for which God, through Christ Jesus, is calling us" (Phil. 3:13–14, NLT). Instead of allowing yourself to become marginalized by the magnification of the rearview mirror, remember Paul's words in 2 Thessalonians 3:3: "But the Lord is faithful, and He will strengthen you and protect you from the evil one" (NASB). You see, Jesus canceled our past with His blood, as my mother so wisely reminds me every chance she gets. "In him we have redemption through his blood, the forgiveness of sins, in accordance with the riches of God's grace" (Eph. 1:7).

What a marvelous gift we have been given! Hang on to it and remember it the next time the demonic shadows of the enemy appear. Don't turn to fear. Turn on the light, turn up the praise, take authority, and apply the blood of Jesus as you remember the words of Psalm 62:6–7: "So why would I let worry paralyze me, even when troubles multiply around me? God's glory is all around me! His wraparound presence is all I need, for the Lord is my Savior, my hero, and my life-giving strength" (TPT).

JUST BREATHE

The Spirit of God has made me; the breath
of the Almighty gives me life.

—JOB 33:4

L IFE IS FULL of seasons of uncertainty, which can turn into seasons of fear when we fail to take hold of God's promises and live in the reality they offer us. Whether you are getting ready to speak on a stage to thousands or simply watching your children walk out the front door, fear can dominate life at times. This was true for me and Pat until we invited the breath of God into our lives at a deeper level. God has given us a promise in Psalm 23:3: "True to your word, you let me catch my breath and send me in the right direction" (MSG). God wants to refresh His children to protect His reputation.

Have you ever been in a situation where you or someone you were with couldn't breathe? If you have, you know it can be very scary. Whatever the issue—whether it be asthma, bronchitis, pneumonia, or COPD—watching someone struggling to breathe creates immediate feelings of extreme helplessness. When our daughter, Abby, was very young, she battled asthma, especially in the fall and winter months. If she caught a cold or any other ailment, it would always trigger an asthma attack. She was placed on a daily inhaled steroid and an emergency inhaler. During that season there were many times she could not catch her breath and the emergency inhaler seemed to be of no help. Those were fearful moments for all of us. Our only recourse was to take her to the hospital, where they would put her on a nebulizer to help her breathe. We can remember saying to her, "Calm down and try to relax, Abby, and just take a deep breath."

Abby was healed of asthma and has not had any issues in many years. When I began to struggle with asthma issues myself, I realized my words of comfort and instruction during Abby's attacks were in reality very difficult for her to accomplish. I was plagued with constant coughing to the point of feeling as though I could not breathe. It was then I realized it is not as simple as just trying to relax and take a deep breath. Fear tries to overtake you when life-giving oxygen is not accessible. That kind of fear only exacerbates an already panicked situation. You become frantic, making your breathing even more erratic. Over time I learned to center myself in the presence of God when I was in the middle of one of those attacks and allow Him to calm my spirit and help me to see past my fear. This became life to me as God's breath would begin to fill my lungs and slow my breathing so I could take in more oxygen.

Have you ever been so frightened that it took your

breath away? One of the first responses to fear is to hold your breath. The problem with holding your breath is when you do, you are not taking in enough oxygen. The lack of oxygen can result in several physical responses such as disorientation, confusion, and loss of balance. Interestingly the same is true in the spiritual when we do not take in enough life-giving breath from God the Father. Daily time in God's presence fills up our spiritual oxygen tanks. Without God's life-giving breath on a regular basis, we become disoriented in our thought processes and lose our balance and focus. When this happens, it is hard to make sound, biblical decisions. In those fight-or-flight moments, God's breath will bring light and life to the situation. In moments of fear it is vitally important to remind ourselves to stop, return to God's presence, and just breathe. As the beloved of God we are created to do more than merely survive. God intends for us to live in the abundance of His presence where fear cannot have the upper hand.

It was during the season of great uncertainty brought on by the leukemia that God began to deal with me on the issue of creating an atmosphere for His breath to flow freely in our lives and our home. Pat and I realized we did not want a mere visitation from God in moments of fear and need. We desired a habitation of the very breath of God. You see, God should never be just a visitor in our lives, allowed entrance only after we put our best image forward for Him. God should be given complete ownership to reside in our lives and our homes as His primary residence. He always has full access to see the good, the bad, and the ugly, so why not give Him full permission through our submission to intervene and take control of every aspect of our lives? Allowing God to fully own your house so you can fully reside in Him enables you to submit fully to His will. In this way we are truly His children under His loving care.

As Pat and I began to experience the habitation of God in our own lives and realized how powerful and life-changing it was, we felt compelled to share it with others. It was out of this journey into the very breath of God that He birthed *The Breathing Room* through us. We created this biweekly Facebook Live stream from our home to encourage others to taste and see the goodness of God in their own lives. We knew that daily encounters with God's breath and power create an atmosphere for the miraculous. In this place of freedom, purpose, and supernatural revelation God moves to bless us. Since we started *The Breathing Room*, we have had as many as fifty thousand views weekly. People from all over the world are creating their own breathing rooms. With fear impacting people worldwide, this powerful message of inviting God to breathe on every aspect of our lives is bringing freedom from fear, anxiety, and discouragement.

When we are faced with fearful and uncertain situations, we must remind ourselves that God's breath gives us life and life abundantly, as stated in Job 33:4: "The Spirit of God has made me; the breath of the Almighty gives me life." In life we do not merely want to survive; we want to truly live in the fullness God has for us. If we allow it, fear can penetrate every area of our lives, even to the point of loss of life-giving breath. Yet the great news for children of God is God wants to breathe new life into us daily, to comfort and strengthen us with the ability to fight the battle against fear. When we are faced with the fight-or-flight response to the enemy, the breath of God gives us the strength to stand firm and fight rather than take flight and run.

THE BREATH OF GOD

Let's talk about the breath of God. It is important to understand the breath of God to realize how it impacts our life and separates us from fear. The world and our very being was formed by the breath of God. Look at Genesis 1:2–3: "The earth was formless and empty, darkness was over the surface of the deep, and the Spirit of God was hovering over the waters. And God said, 'Let there be light.'" This scripture is so powerful! God *said*. God spoke, and breath went forth. He said, "Let there be light," and there was light! Words take form through breath. God spoke, breath came forth, and what God spoke was formed!

If we just use the English word *spirit*, we will miss what is being described in Genesis 1. The Bible is describing a scenario where breath is involved—the breath of God. The word *spirit* in the Hebrew is *ruwach*, which is often translated "wind" or "breath."[1] The Greek word translated "Spirit" is *pneuma*, which means air in motion, wind, or breath.[2] Knowing the meaning of *Spirit*, we can safely translate and understand Genesis 1:2–3 in this manner: "The earth was formless and empty, darkness was over the surface of the deep, and the Spirit [breath] of God was hovering over the waters, and God spoke [or breathed] and there was light!" He breathed, and His breath lit up the heavens and the earth. His very essence lights up every dark place. God's Spirit, or breath, always brings life!

Think about the last time you felt as though fear had taken your breath away. Think about when you felt anxiety over an important task. Maybe you have feared failing or being inadequate. Have you ever been overwhelmed by fear of tragedies taking place throughout the world? Have you ever experienced fear that your future was uncertain? The apostle Paul strongly believed in the Word of God's ability to strengthen, guide, and teach us all we need to stay the course and walk in faith. The Bible contains two letters Paul addressed directly to his protégé Timothy. In chapter 3 we discussed one of those letters, which specifically describes how to defeat fear. Paul wrote that letter during a period in history when Christians were being persecuted in cruel and torturous ways. But this letter contained even more guidance for Timothy. Paul wrote in 2 Timothy 3:14, "Continue in what you have learned and have become convinced of, because you know those from whom you learned it."

In writing those words, Paul acknowledged his realization he would not be around much longer to lead and guide Timothy. He wanted to be absolutely certain Timothy knew where his strength came from, how to defeat fear, and where life would come from when it seemed trials and tribulations would cause him to become weary and out of breath. It is no wonder that this letter included a powerful truth and source of encouragement. Paul reminded Timothy of God's breath. He told Timothy that *all* Scripture was God-breathed. That is why when we feed on the Word and digest every part of it, we will never be out of breath or out of life.

Let's jump down to 2 Timothy 3:16: "All scripture is God-breathed and is useful for teaching, rebuking, correcting and training in righteousness." The word *God-breathed* is *theopneustos* in the Greek.[3] It directly relates to God's Spirit, or *pneuma*, which we know can also be translated "breath." This is the only place in Scripture where we find this particular word *theopneustos*. However, it is definitely not the only place where we find the image of God breathing. We see God breathe life into the nostrils of man in Genesis 2:7: "Then the LORD God formed a man from the dust of the ground and breathed into his nostrils the breath of life, and the man became a living being." Without the actual breath of God, we cannot truly live. We were created to protect the breath of God in our lives. Fear is a means by which Satan intends to rob us of life.

Let's revisit Genesis 2:7 to see how God created each of us for a purpose. Look at the creation of man. The Bible says that God breathed into the nostrils of Adam. This is the beginning of mankind. But what about Eve? The Bible does not use the same terminology (God breathed) when describing the creation of Eve. This is in no way an indication that women are less valuable. It actually is a testament to how important women are. It is a simple statement that was left out, and I have concluded that it was on purpose.

Look at how God created Eve in Genesis 2:22, "Then the LORD God made a woman from the rib he had taken out of the man, and he brought her to the man." I fully understand that it can be assumed God would have naturally breathed into Eve as He did with Adam. However, I searched every translation, and it is not what God thought was the most important thing for us to know about the creation of Eve. He had already breathed life into mankind. However, I think He felt it important for us to know the magnitude and the importance of the breath that was given to us.

Look what God chose to create woman out of. He didn't use the femur, or thighbone, symbolizing we were created to walk side by side. God chose the rib. There is significance to God's use of the rib that relates to both what the rib is designed for in the natural and its purpose in our spiritual life. The functions of the ribs include respiration and protection. The rib cage facilitates breathing by expanding and contracting as we inhale and exhale. The ribs protect vital organs necessary to sustain life, including the heart, lungs, liver, and kidneys.[4]

I hope you are beginning to realize everything in Scripture is put there for a reason and leads us to a greater understanding of our relationship with God. The question is, How willing are we to dig into God's Word to find that revelation? God is purposeful in all He does to rescue us and prepare us for any and all attacks from the enemy. He chose to create woman out of the very bone that protects the heart, liver, kidneys, and lungs.

Let's look at how that relates to the spiritual purpose of God's use of the rib. We accept Christ into our hearts, and if Christ lives in us, then we are carrying the revival fire of God everywhere we go. In the natural our liver and kidneys filter out all of the impurities that could harm us.

Our lungs house the very breath given to us as a source of life and life more abundantly. God breathed life into mankind and then stressed how important the breath of God is by forming woman out of the very thing that was needed to protect it in our natural lives.

The spiritual parallel is that we must protect the breath of God in our own lives, in the lives of our families, and in the body of Christ. We are to keep the flame burning and not let the light go out so a lost and dying world can walk away from fear and into the very light and presence of God! This is how the enemy and his weapon of fear are cast out and we are set free. First John 4 tells us, "Perfect love casts out fear" (v. 18, NASB), and "God is love" (v. 16). And we read in John 1:1, "In the beginning was the Word, and the Word was with God, and the Word was God." God is love, and God is the Word. His breath spoke the world into existence. This is why perfect love casts out fear—God's very breath blows it out for us!

EQUIPPED TO BE BOLD

This same breath of God is also demonstrated in Acts 4:31: "And when they had prayed, the place where they were assembled together was shaken; and they were all filled with the Holy Spirit, and they spoke the word of God with *boldness*" (NKJV, emphasis added). Again, the word *Spirit* is the Greek word *pneuma*, which is God's breath. Did you catch what was stated? When they prayed (spent time with God), God's Spirit (His breath) filled them, and the result was a boldness they did not possess before being breathed upon. Fear is the thief of boldness, but the breath of God breaks through fear and equips us to be bold.

Before God breathed on the disciples, they were a bunch of misfit nobodies. It was His breath that made them heroes of the faith and paved the way for Christians around the world today. This small group of people changed history after they were filled with God's breath. They were hiding in an upper room for fear of man until God made them bold by breathing upon them. He will breathe upon us in the same way today, giving us boldness to withstand any trial.

There are very few sounds as beautiful as the sound of a newborn baby crying in announcement of his grand entrance into the world. Why does a baby cry when he is born? Even though there are scientific explanations for this, I like to believe the baby is giving thanks to God with the breath given to bring him life. In that first moment when oxygen fills a newborn's lungs, that baby is declaring to the world, "I made it!" This birth cry is a victory shout, acknowledging the One who breathes life into all creation, the One who brings the breath of protection and deliverance to all who will receive it. We should create an atmosphere where the breath of God flows freely at all times in our lives!

I believe God is about to give CPR to some of you reading this today. You have been gasping for air and reaching for your spiritual inhaler for too long. It's time to take a deep breath and breathe in the life that God has given you. This life is designed to be lived free of fear and instead full of the roar of the Lion of the tribe of Judah. If you feel out of breath today and are struggling to see past the darkness that has overtaken you, I encourage you to receive God's breath. Romans 8:11 tells us, "Yes, God raised Jesus to life! And since God's Spirit of Resurrection lives in you, he will also raise your dying body to life by the same Spirit that breathes life into you!" (TPT). Fear is defeated through the breath of God. Just breathe!

FIVE TRUTHS CONCERNING THE BREATH OF GOD

God's breath gives life.

> The Spirit of God has made me; the breath of the Almighty gives me life.
>
> —JOB 33:4

> By the word of the LORD the heavens were made, and by the breath of His mouth all their host.
>
> —PSALM 33:6, NASB

God's breath breaks the spirit of fear.

> By His breath the heavens are cleared; His hand has pierced the fleeing serpent.
>
> —JOB 26:13, NASB

God's breath drives out darkness.

> The earth was formless and empty, darkness was over the surface of the deep, and the Spirit of God was hovering over the waters. And God said, "Let there be light," and there was light.
>
> GENESIS 1:2–3

God's breath brings understanding.

> But it is a spirit in man, and the breath of the Almighty gives them understanding.
>
> —JOB 32:8, NASB

God's breath heals our dry bones.

> Thus says the Lord GOD to these bones, "Behold, I will cause breath to enter you that you may come to life."
>
> —EZEKIEL 37:5, NASB

CHAPTER 5

COURAGE, IT'S ME!

Peter, suddenly bold, said, "Master, if it's really you,
call me to come to you on the water." He said, "Come
ahead." Jumping out of the boat, Peter walked on
the water to Jesus. But when he looked down at the
waves churning beneath his feet, he lost his nerve
and started to sink. He cried, "Master, save me!" Jesus
did not hesitate. He reached down and grabbed his
hand. Then he said, "Faint-heart, what got into you?"

—MATTHEW 14:28–31, MSG

I (KAREN) HAVE A confession to make. Fear has been my nemesis the majority of my life. It was with me as a child, as a teenager, and through a portion of my adult life. It traveled with as me as I ministered all over the world. It caused me to wear a mask that hid the torment and misery I felt at times. It caused me to shrink back in crowded rooms when I should have stepped forward. It often delayed my destiny and even shrouded my potential. That nemesis' name is fear! Fear is the figment of the enemy lurking around every corner waiting to pounce. I have learned that walking in my

God-given destiny requires confronting the phantom of my opera! It is a choice each one of us has to make. Proverbs 11:19 says, "Take your stand with God's loyal community and live, or chase after phantoms of evil and die" (MSG).

Just thinking about confronting your fears is often scarier than actually doing it. Yet when you are bold enough to confront what has you by the tail, God will have you minister to others facing the very thing that tried to destroy you. I have always wanted to be a beautiful, majestic, soaring eagle, but more often than not I have felt like a chicken. Over the years I have come to realize that is exactly how the enemy wants me to feel. That is not how God wants me to think, though. He created me to soar like a mighty warrior. I know this because the Bible instructs me to "put on the full armor of God, so that [I] can take [my] stand against the devil's schemes" (Eph. 6:11). Attacks of the enemy are going to come as we walk hand in hand with God. It's up to us to know the weapons of our warfare, to know that God gives us the ability to be warriors and equips us with spiritual armor specifically crafted to bring us victory.

STAND FIRM

The Bible actually says that at times merely standing firm is all it takes to defeat Satan. Ephesians 6:13–14 says, "Therefore put on the full armor of God, so that when the day of evil comes, you may be able to stand your ground, and after you have done everything, to stand. Stand firm then." So many believers don't know how to stand. They are bound and enslaved by a spirit of fear. Fear has the ability to cause our hearts to grow faint and cause us to give up when we have no answers. If we stay bound long enough, we begin to accept fear as a part of life and settle for less than God has for us. Fear of the unknown causes us to lose our sense of adventure and to hold back, doubting our self-worth and our purpose. However, as believers we can turn fear around so the dark, unknown place that has impeded our progress becomes the place where our greatest trust in God is birthed.

God wants to restore our faint hearts. He wants to restore the roar inside us. Fear creates a faint heart, but God wants to strengthen our heart and turn us into lionhearts! Christ died to release us from spiritual slavery. "It is for freedom that Christ has set us free. Stand firm, then, and do not let yourselves be burdened again by a yoke of slavery" (Gal. 5:1). Christians should not be the most fearful creatures on the planet. We have a powerful, loving heavenly Father who has equipped us well for battle. "So you have not received a spirit that makes you fearful slaves. Instead, you received God's Spirit when he adopted you as his own children. Now we call him, 'Abba, Father'" (Rom. 8:15, NLT).

How sad it is that Satan believes in our purpose more than we do. He is not concerned about who we have been but who we were created to be. The battle is real. Satan's hope is that if he can keep the blinders of fear over our eyes, we will never be the warriors God created us to be. The devil is a liar (John 8:44) and a thief who comes only to steal, kill, and destroy (John 10:10). Yet we have Jesus, who comes that we may have life and have it to the full. Because of His finished work on the cross, we now have His Holy Spirit to equip us. We have armor to ensure our victory.

> Stand firm then, with the belt of truth buckled around your waist, with the breastplate of righteousness in place, and with your feet fitted with the readiness that comes from the gospel of peace, in addition to all this, take up the shield of faith, with which you can extinguish the flaming arrows of the evil one. Take the helmet of salvation and the sword of the spirit, which is the word of God.
> —Ephesians 6:14–17

Each part of our armor is designed to defeat the enemy's onslaught of fear. We have the belt of truth to know that God's Word is trustworthy and true. This belt is the first part of the armor mentioned because God wants us to know that we can have full confidence in every single thing He says. We can trust Him to keep us safe in the midst of battle.

He has given us a breastplate of righteousness to protect our hearts, and the weapon of love so fear cannot take root and weaken our spirit with doubt. He has fitted our feet with the readiness that comes from His peace, because when we are at peace in the knowledge of His security, we can run to the battle rather than away from it. We are equipped to charge forth and take back the ground that was stolen from us.

God has given us a shield of faith so that we can call those things that are not as though they were (Rom. 4:17) in order to dodge every flaming arrow of the enemy, and a helmet of salvation to protect our sound mind from illogical, unfounded, and absurd thoughts. And let us not forget the most powerful part of our armor, the sword of the Spirit, the very breath of God, which can create and destroy with one single word.

The question for you and me as believers is, What will you do with what God has equipped you with? Will you step out boldly and confidently, taking up God's weapons of warfare, and confront the liar? Will you declare from somewhere beneath the layers of insecurity that you were born for such a time as this? Somewhere beneath the shy exterior is a declarer of truth! Somewhere between "I can't" and "I must" is a warrior preparing for battle! Somewhere between what others have said and what God has declared is a freedom fighter! Somewhere between "I am stepping out," and "Oh no, I'm about to drown" is a hero of faith. To understand this better, let's look at a passage from Matthew.

> Peter, suddenly bold, said, "Master, if it's really you, call me to come to you on the water."
>
> He said, "Come ahead."
>
> Jumping out of the boat, Peter walked on the water to Jesus. But when he looked down at the waves churning beneath his feet, he lost his nerve and started to sink. He cried, "Master, save me!"
>
> Jesus didn't hesitate. He reached down and grabbed his hand. Then he said, "Faint-heart, what got into you?
>
> —Matthew 14:28–31, msg

This man, who would become one of the great leaders of the church, this Simon Peter, stepped boldly out of the boat and then began to sink in fear. This big, tough fisherman began sinking in waves of despair. Wait a minute! Isn't this the same Simon Peter who preached so boldly on the day of Pentecost? (See Acts 2:14–17.) Isn't this the same Simon Peter whose shadow healed the sick? (See Acts 5:15.) Yes, it is! Peter illustrates an important spiritual principle— that a lion sometimes acts like a lamb just before it roars. In other words, our timid behavior isn't our true identity. We may act like a lamb as the battle looms, but when we pick up God's weapons of warfare, we become lions. Peter was timid at that moment on the water, but he would not remain timid. That rough-hewn fisherman from the shores of the Sea of Galilee would go on to become a leader in the fledgling Christian church, forever shaping history according to God's plan. In fact, Jesus declared Peter the rock on which He would build His church.

The name Peter is the Greek term *Petros*, which means rock.[1] When Peter proclaimed Jesus was the Messiah, Jesus said of Peter's faith, "God bless you, Simon, son of Jonah! You didn't get that answer out of books or from teachers. My Father in heaven, God himself, let you in on this secret of who I really am. And now I'm going to tell you who you are, *really* are. You are Peter, a rock. This is the rock on which I will put together my church, a church so expansive with energy that not even the gates of hell will be able to keep it out" (Matt. 16:18, MSG). Not only would Simon Peter be the rock on which the church would be built, he was the first apostle named in the lists of Jesus' twelve disciples.[2] Martyred for Christ, Peter was crucified in Rome under Emperor Nero, and church tradition claims he asked to be turned upside down because he said he was not worthy to be crucified in the same manner as his beloved Savior.[3]

CONFRONT FEAR

I hope you can see yourself as God sees you. I pray you are beginning to feel the roar He has placed inside of you as you arise out of the darkness. Very rarely do we become who we were created to be without a fight. It is your time to fight. It is your time to love the sound of your feet walking away from those things that do not belong to you. So often we wake up to the enemy taunting and intimidating us. Many times fear of failure, fear of what people think, or even fear of losing control can make us strive too hard for perfection. Since there is none who is perfect except Jesus, this kind of fearful thinking sets us up for disappointment and failure. We cannot attain perfection until the day we are finally with our Savior. "And I am certain that God, who began the good work within you, will continue his work until it is finally finished on the day when Christ Jesus returns" (Phil. 1:6, NLT). You were born to be real, not perfect.

I used to think the things I walked through made me who I am. But then one of my dear spiritual fathers, Pastor George Sawyer, said, "Karen, your issues do not make you; they reveal you." Whoa! How true are those words! Think of Peter's denying Jesus three times. God had to reveal to Peter who he was in order to reveal to Peter who He created him to be. It's what comes out of our cups when we are bumped, what overflows out of our lives in the worst of times, that reveals who we really are. It takes courage to be great. It takes faith to believe God is who He says He is, to believe that He is the same yesterday, today, and tomorrow. Every situation where the enemy tries to place fear and doubt in your life actually reveals what is already inside of you.

Confronting fear always starts in your night season. In Matthew 14:23–26, the disciples were afraid because they had misplaced Jesus in their night season. They were in the boat, heading to the other side without Jesus. He had gone up on a mountainside by Himself to pray. When He did come to them, in the fourth watch of the night, He came walking on the water. Awakened from their sleep by His supernatural presence, fear set in because they thought Jesus was a ghost, not their beloved friend. Their fear, their perceived aberration, grew into an absolute.

How often do we let this very thing happen in our own lives? When life is chugging along smoothly, we put Jesus on a shelf or somewhere in the depths of our hearts and minds. Then when a crisis comes, we cry out in fear because we have misplaced our Savior. We have to scramble around, trying to remember where we last felt His presence in our lives. Jesus never leaves us or forsakes us. He is always right where we left off in our relationship. If you don't feel Him close by, it's time to retrace your steps and remember where you were when you walked away and stopped spending time with Him. Never negotiate your anointing away because you do not believe Jesus is close by.

Our tendency to leave Jesus behind is why we need to

nurture and cultivate our spiritual senses every day by spending time with our loving Savior, in the good times and in the bad times. Time spent daily in His presence means we don't have to worry or fret, because we know exactly where God is—right beside us every day.

> Don't fret or worry. Instead of worrying, pray. Let petitions and praises shape your worries into prayers, letting God know your concerns. Before you know it, a sense of God's wholeness, everything coming together for good, will come and settle you down. It's wonderful what happens when Christ displaces worry at the center of your life.
> —Philippians 4:6–7, MSG

Before going up on the mountain alone to pray, Jesus told the disciples to go to the other side. He had not changed His mind. God doesn't change His mind. Often, when things are not happening the way we want them to or as quickly as we would like them to, we think God has changed His mind. If we are in a frightening or uncomfortable situation, then God must have changed His mind, right? Sometimes the process to our promise and our freedom takes perseverance and patience. Sometimes our freedom is a process that requires change and contending, not giving up but believing without seeing. This process often requires total trust and a total abandonment of self. God's Word is true and just. He does not change His mind. (See James 1:17.) We change, but God does not change. He is the same yesterday, today, and forever. If God says He will meet you on the other side of your situation, you better believe you will make it there in victory. Jesus promised in Matthew 11:28, "Come to me, all you who are weary and burdened, and I will give you rest." He has not changed His mind.

Nighttime had come, and the disciples were floating in the dark, comfortable and satisfied with what had taken place on the hillside, comfortable enough to misplace their Lord. Jesus, on the other hand, was neither comfortable nor satisfied. John the Baptist had just been beheaded and Jesus had just fed five thousand. He needed to go and meet with the Father. Have you ever noticed from Scripture that Jesus never put His Father on the shelf? He always did quite the opposite. He constantly went to the Father, to be with Him, to feel His heartbeat, to receive His breath. We must not become comfortable and satisfied in moments when life seems easy. That is the time to press in for more of God, to cry out for more of God. The mundane can be the seductress that thwarts the supernatural. It's in the mundane, in the comfortable, that we misplace Jesus so He is no longer at the center of our lives.

When Jesus finished praying, He went to join the disciples. The boat was far away from the shore at that point, so Jesus decided to walk on the water to get to the boat. Wow! Here was their Lord walking on the water! Yet the disciples were so wrapped up in their false perceptions that they missed a moment to celebrate the laws of nature being broken. They were witnessing the supernatural of God and perceived it as something ungodly. How often do we miss the supernatural intervention of God because of overwhelming fear and anxiety that blinds us to His reality? Jesus interrupts the natural with the supernatural in our lives on a regular basis, but we tend to focus on the crisis instead of the miracle. Perhaps that is because we become so exhausted by life that we allow our focus to shift from God's truths to Satan's lies. Whatever the reason, we must develop the habit of always adjusting our focus so as to keep our eyes on Jesus, the One who walks on what tries to take us out. Jesus stands over every ocean of darkness. He walks upon whatever wants to drown you. (See Genesis 1:2.)

FIND YOUR COURAGE

When the disciples saw what they thought was a ghost approaching them on the water, they gave in to fear. Jesus, seeing how frightened they were, was quick to comfort them, saying, "Courage, it's me. Don't be afraid" (Matt. 14:27, MSG). I hope by the time you are finished reading this chapter, you are standing up and shouting and declaring, "Courage, it's me!" Don't you love the way that sounds? It's as if you are reminding your courage who you have been in the past, as if you are calling forth the courage God placed inside of you.

This past year, while battling the diagnosis of leukemia, there were days I needed to be reminded there was courage in me. There were days I woke up and I didn't feel well, when my joints ached and my head hurt and I didn't feel very strong. On those days, I didn't want to get up and get going. I wanted to sulk and feel sorry for myself. On those days I had a decision to make. I could either be a fearful quitter, or I could take up the armor and stand. I am not a quitter. On those days when the enemy tried to come against me, I rose up in defiance and attacked him because I wasn't going down without a fight.

I chose to get up, walk to the bathroom, and look in the mirror, remembering Matthew 14:27, when the enemy tried to make the disciples think Jesus was a ghost on the water and not their rescuer and deliverer. The enemy will always distort the truth. Cancer is a distortion of God's truth. On those mornings, as I looked in the mirror, I declared leukemia a distortion, an aberration. Instead of seeing what the enemy wanted me to see—someone tired and achy and feeling weak—I was going to see what God saw in me—a warrior, dressed for battle. I would literally stand in front of the mirror and make courageous declarations.

> Courage, it's me! It's me! *No fear!* I may not see you, but I know you are there, courage! Arise and show yourself!

> God is my strength, and in Him I trust! I believe what he says in Isaiah 41:13, "For I am the LORD your God, who takes hold of your right hand and says to you, Do not fear; I will help you."

> If God says there is courage in me, then there is courage! And this fear is courage waiting to be awakened!

My battle cries brought me peace in the darkest of times. They gave me strength when I was weak, courage when I was fearful. My ocean of despair did not compare to His ocean of love. God loves us enough to meet us right where we are and walk us to safety. Whatever you are walking through, you can rest in the knowledge that God is working in your family. He is working on your kids, your health, and your situation. He is interrupting the laws of nature for you! He will not abandon you.

> Don't be afraid, I've redeemed you. I've called your name. You're mine. When you're in over your head, I'll be there with you. When you're in rough waters, you will not go down. When you're between a rock and a hard place, it won't be a dead end—because I am God, your personal God.
> —ISAIAH 43:1–3, MSG

What the devil meant for evil, God will use for your good. Remember what Joseph said to his brothers? "You intended to harm me, but God intended it for good to accomplish what is now being done, the saving of many lives" (Gen. 50:20). God is not the one coming against you. The devil is our adversary. Don't measure the goodness of God according to your résumé of pain. Quit cursing what you don't understand and ask God to give you spiritual eyes to see Him in the midst of your situation according to Scripture. (See Ephesians 1:18.)

God wants you to awaken and see your battle in the spirit realm. Open your spiritual eyes! Satan is at war with your future courage. Fear is like spiritual blinders. If the enemy can blind you with fear, you won't be able to see the victory right in front of you. Fear will try to become your compass, leading you away from God and His truths. Don't let fear guide you in the wrong direction. When you are led by the Spirit, you are always led into truth (John 16:13). Allow God's Spirit to become your compass and your GPS (God Positioning System).

I want to remind you today that if God called you out, He will meet you at your point of doubt. Simon Peter went from being bold to losing his nerve in a matter of minutes. What I love is that Jesus was not taken aback by Peter's fear or the fact that he started out so strong and then allowed the waves to distract him. Jesus saw the fear in Peter before he even stepped out of the boat. He knew what was about to happen, but He also knew that Peter was about to learn something very important about faith and trust—that it's not about the waves. It's not about the fear. It's not about the pain or the situation. It's about the relationship—knowing who Jesus is and knowing that in Him there is no fear. In Christ there is no reason for doubt or concern. Jesus is our very source of strength and courage. Peter needed to know this, to learn this through experience in order to stand as a rock on which God would build His church. The wind and the waves will come. You will experience a rough time in night seasons. That is why we need to learn what Peter had to learn—to keep our eyes on Jesus no matter what. He will always be there for us, not to condemn but to speak to our hearts and lovingly say, "Faintheart, what got into you?"

The beating of your heart will always grow faint when God's heart is not intertwined with yours, when your affections and your passions don't match His heart. We are living in the day of fainthearts. The enemy is wearing out those who are supposed to be strong and bold. I don't want to be a faintheart. I want to be a lionheart! Peter allowed the chaos around him to make him forget who called him out. He was fainthearted, but not forever. Just look at what happened when Jesus took Peter by the hand. "The two of them climbed into the boat, and the wind died down. The disciples in the boat, having watched the whole thing, worshiped Jesus, saying, 'This is it! You are God's Son for sure!'" (Matt. 14:32–33, MSG). Peter's faith got him onto the water, but then the hand of God led him back into the place of safety.

So often we think that because we have moments of weakness, failure, and doubt, God can't use us, so we give up. We think that because we react with fear or anxiety to difficult situations, we are somehow disqualified. The reality is the enemy wants those situations to disqualify and deter our purpose and our destiny. That's the lie. The truth is those situations are opportunities to let courage arise and to get back up and choose to see the truth standing right in front of us. People are watching to see how you navigate your night seasons. You can be the revelation of who they can become. I know this to be true because I walked it out daily. Every morning the enemy wanted me to see the lie of cancer when I looked in the mirror. I chose to see courage instead. God did not give me the cancer, but He definitely used it to stretch me and to awaken courage inside of me until I became a thorn in the enemy's side.

Once you find your courage and your lion's roar, the devil is the one who gets afraid because God will use the very thing Satan tried to kill you with as a weapon to defeat him. One moment Satan thought that he had humiliated Peter. But in the next moment Jesus showed Peter and the disciples exactly who He was. The devil wanted to separate

Peter and the disciples from the Lord because he knew that once God's courage was awakened in them, they were unstoppable. Peter jumped out of the boat with zeal and passion, proceeded to sink with fear and trembling, and was rescued and restored by the Son of God! In a moment the schemes of the enemy were thwarted as the plans of God were put in place.

> But one thing I do: Forgetting what is behind and straining toward what is ahead, I press on toward the goal to win the prize for which God has called me heavenward in Christ Jesus.
>
> —PHILIPPIANS 3:13–14

It's time for you to step out! God is about to meet you in your sinking! He is about to grab your hand and pull you up out of the crashing waves of life and the darkness that has surrounded you! Be assured—He *will* reach out and not hesitate. He *will* reveal courage in you and then take you back to the boat where the others are watching, where your family and friends are watching and searching for courage in their own fear. Your courage will bring hope and life to those who are lost and in a prison of fear. Remember what was said about Jesus in Isaiah 53:7, "He was oppressed and afflicted, yet he did not open his mouth; he was led like a lamb to the slaughter, and as a sheep before its shearers is silent, so he did not open his mouth."

The Lion always acts like a lamb right before He roars! Jesus was the Lamb who became the Lion when He roared from the cross, "It is finished!" Jesus defeated Satan and took back the keys to death, hell, and the grave so that He could give us power, love, and a sound mind. (See 2 Timothy 1:7.) Peter would go from the moment on the lake with Jesus to become the rock on which the church would be built, leading with boldness and authority.

Have the cares and concerns and worries of life caused you to become fainthearted? If so, take heart! God understands, and He won't leave you in the night season. He is reaching out to you right now without hesitation. He is calling to you, saying, "Faintheart, what got into you? Arise, and step out of the chaos of the crashing waves and lies of the enemy. Take My hand today and declare, 'Courage, it's me! I won't be afraid.'"

If you stepped out on the water and took your eyes off of Jesus, just reach out and take His hand, and He will lead you back to safety. He will make you a witness to all those watching that not only did He rescue you, but also He is indeed the Son of God. Be the example of who others can become. Have courage! Arise! Don't look at the failures of the past. Look to the future with courage. "You can't go back and make a new start, but you can start right now and make a brand new ending."[4]

CHAPTER 7

PEACE IN THE STORM

The LORD gives strength to his people; the
LORD blesses his people with peace.
—PSALM 29:11

TODAY, I (KAREN) am reminded of the beach as I write. Maybe that is because it is winter and the shorter, dreary, cold days have me yearning for longer days and sunny skies when I can soak up all the vitamin D the sun has to offer and be mesmerized by the sound of the ocean crashing against the shore. Whatever the reason, the beach is definitely my happy place. There is something special about the sound and view of the ocean that causes me to lean in a little closer and listen for God to speak. Perhaps it is because in that environment I can tune out the chaos of the hectic schedule we keep and actually listen.

As I sit and think of this beautiful, calm, peaceful scene and the methodical movement of such a massive body of water, I am keenly aware the seas are not always so calm. Storms are inevitable, and what seems so peaceful can quickly turn to chaos and danger, and disrupt what was once so beautiful and peaceful. It reminds me of our seasons of rest and peace that so often get interrupted and disturbed by the enemy's attacks. Satan brings spiritual storms into our lives in an attempt to rob us of the peace we have in Christ. Just as we have to pay attention to the weather patterns when planning our retreats to the beach, so must we stay alert to the enemy's schemes to be prepared for the storms he brings. One of the ways we can do this is to listen for God to speak in the busyness of our lives.

Let me ask you, Has the thief called fear stolen your peace? Are you afraid and in a storm right now, struggling to hear God's voice above the wind, the thunder, the flying debris, and the waves crashing all around you? Have you ever longed for peace in the midst of turmoil and worry, or searched for joy in the midst of sorrow and pain? If you answered yes to any of those questions, then this chapter is for you. As you read, be prepared for the overwhelming love and peace of God to fill your life as you experience the breath and power of God's presence. I want you to know that it is completely possible for you to be at total peace in the midst of your storm. In fact not only is it possible, but it is also God's desire and plan that you be at peace. My prayer for you today is Numbers 6:26, "May the LORD show you his favor and give you his peace" (NLT). I challenge you to take a few moments to praise and worship God right now for who He is and welcome Him into your storm today.

BUSYNESS IS NOT A SPIRITUAL GIFT

In the middle of the season of the cancer diagnosis, one of the things God spoke to me about was the fact that I was running way too hard and staying way too busy. A big part of me felt as if I would stay physically stronger if I stayed busy at God's work, as if taking time to rest was somehow less spiritual and weak. Quite the opposite is true. God intends for us to have times of rest to renew our strength. When I was diagnosed with leukemia, I decided I would work, work, work, and never give in or slow down. That was my defiant stance toward the enemy. While staying busy definitely helped keep my mind off the cancer diagnosis, my overboard activity led to extreme exhaustion. Pat would constantly tell me to take time to rest, but I was just plain angry at the devil and pushed harder to prove I was strong and the devil was wrong.

One morning in my prayer time God spoke to my spirit and said, "Karen, busyness is not a spiritual gift! It's in the resting that you slow down enough to listen for My voice. I want to speak to you during this storm." Are you in the middle of a storm that has left you floundering to find your peace? Floundering to catch your breath? Floundering at the deafening sound of your heart beating out of your chest in fear and panic? If so, I pray you slow down enough to listen for the voice of God. He wants to speak peace to your storm today. Just listen, and you will hear Him guiding and directing you to the safety of the shore. God has always spoken. He spoke the world into existence and light into the darkness in Genesis. He spoke life into mankind and spoke to Adam and Eve as He walked with them in the cool of the evening in the garden. You need to know that God still speaks! He did not stop speaking to His children when the last book of the Bible was written. He is speaking to you. Will you listen?

There is something else important to understand about listening to the voice of God. So often when He speaks to us in the midst of our stormy circumstances, it is not our circumstances that change as much as it is we who change as a result of hearing His voice. Let's look at a few instances of this from Scripture. In Exodus 20 God spoke to Moses on Mount Sinai, giving him the Ten Commandments. When Moses came down from the mountain, the Israelites were behaving as badly as ever—worse in fact. In frustration and anger Moses threw the tablets to the ground, breaking them. Things continued to go poorly. Moses was in the middle of his storm. Then Moses went into the tent of meeting to meet with the Lord. There in the tent, the place of meeting, God spoke to Moses: "My Presence will go with you, and I will give you rest" (Exod. 33:14). From that place of rest the storm began to subside. It subsided because Moses was reacting to the storm in a different way—from a place of rest where he could hear the voice of the Lord.

God spoke to Elijah in the cave in 1 Kings 19, bringing peace to his fear and speaking destiny and purpose into his life. God spoke to Hosea at an auction, telling him to love his bride, even though she would be unfaithful, as an example of how He loves us even though we run away to our own pleasures. God spoke to David as he gathered five stones and strengthened him with courage to kill Goliath, the giant in his way. God spoke to Simeon as he held a baby who would become our Deliverer. Nicodemus went looking for God in the night and found Jesus, who taught him about believing beyond the natural as well as understanding and seeing beyond our carnal eyesight. God spoke to the Samaritan woman at the well, bringing kingdom life and light to her broken life. He met her where she was, told her the reality of her life, and then offered her a solution for her thirst that could not be quenched by earthly means.

I hope you see that in every situation peace entered the situation when God spoke. The situation didn't necessarily change, but the person did when he heard God's voice and received His peace. When we allow peace to walk in, everything changes. In our loneliness, fear, and despair—in our storm—everything in us will change when God walks in. When we slow down long enough to listen for His voice, His very breath will bring peace and calm and clarity. I know this to be true because God definitely speaks to me!

He spoke to me on a park bench when I was thirteen to let me know I was never alone, He saw me, and He knew my name. He spoke to me in my season of desperation in wanting another child by giving me a vision of China and my daughter waiting for us to get there to bring her home. God spoke to me in the thunder in the night to write the book *Dehydrated* so others would know there is hope for their dry and weary lives. He spoke to me to get up at five o'clock every morning for a season, beckoning me to Psalm 27:8: "My heart has heard you say, 'Come and talk with me.' And my heart responds, 'LORD, I am coming'"

(NLT). God spoke to me at my kitchen sink when He asked me, "Karen, do you trust Me?"

God's voice prepared me for the cancer storm that would disrupt our lives. Even in that storm His voice, His breath, filled my lungs with the ability to praise Him. In that place of praise I was able to receive His overflowing peace to sustain me until I reached the shore safely. When we are faced with fear of the storms that rage, we have two options. We can walk away and be tossed about and shaken, or we can dive in and be made whole in God's peace. When His breath fills my lungs, I can finally breathe again. When He speaks, my countenance changes, not just my situation. "When Moses came down from Mount Sinai with the two tablets of the covenant law in his hands, he was not aware that his face was radiant because he had spoken with the LORD" (Exod. 34:29).

Talking with God changed Moses' very appearance and his countenance—so much so that the people recognized Moses was different and were afraid to go near him. When you get free, people won't understand. They will always want you to go back to the person who doesn't expose the fact that they need freedom as well. It is not what you go through that matters; it is whom you walk through it with and whom you talk with in the midst of it that matters. You change when you listen for God's voice. God wants us to draw close and listen. He desires to spend time with us and give us revelation of who He is and who He is calling us to be. It is God's voice and His breath that fills our space and changes our perception of our storms.

GOD NEVER STOPS SPEAKING TO US

Some of you may feel as if the heavens are silent or that you are not worthy of God speaking to you. Look at the people God spoke to in the Bible. Not many were worthy. Not many were high society. Not many deserved to be spoken to by God. They simply listened, and God transformed them to impact the world. If God seems to be quiet right now, maybe you didn't respond to Him the last time He spoke to you. If God seems distant or standoffish, maybe He is waiting on you to change your stance and sit down and have a conversation with Him.

Matthew 28:20 declares that He is not going anywhere: "And surely I am with you always, to the very end of the age." God tells us that if we talk with Him and cry out to Him, He will answer us. He will speak to us and give us the answers we are looking for. "Call to me and I will answer you and tell you great and unsearchable things you do not know" (Jer. 33:3). God never stops speaking to us. If you are not hearing His voice, could it be that you are just too busy to listen? Jesus said many times in the Gospels, "Whoever has ears, let them hear" (e.g., Matt. 13:9). Many times the church is walking around with deaf ears, waiting for God to use sign language (Give me a sign, God!), but God is saying, "You don't need a sign, but I'll give you a whisper."

Only regular times of prayer with God can provide the essential foundation of our search for greater peace. Trying to become peaceful without spending time with God in prayer is a logical impossibility. Peace can only come from being in regular communion with Him. We need to understand that we can hear God speak in order to fully understand that His voice brings peace to the fear that tries to imprison us. God is the source of all peace. Your peace does not have to vanish in the midst of the storm. In fact the storm is where you can find God's peace! "'Though the mountains be shaken and the hills be removed, yet my unfailing love for you will not be shaken nor my covenant of peace be removed,' says the LORD, who has compassion on you" (Isa. 54:10). Look at what He is saying here. Not only does God give you peace in the storm, but He also has compassion on you!

THE STORM IS TO DISTRACT YOU FROM YOUR MIRACLE

To better understand the peace that comes from hearing God speak, I invite you to take a few minutes and read a passage from the Gospel of Mark. It is a long passage; however, it is a perfect example of God speaking peace into our storms.

> That day when evening came, he said to his disciples, "Let us go over to the other side." Leaving the crowd behind, they took him along, just as he was, in the boat. There were also other boats with him. A furious squall came up, and the waves broke over the boat, so that it was nearly swamped. Jesus was in the stern, sleeping on a cushion. The disciples woke him and said to him, "Teacher, don't you care if we drown?"
> He got up, rebuked the wind and said to the

waves, "Quiet! Be still!" Then the wind died down and it was completely calm.

He said to his disciples, "Why are you so afraid? Do you still have no faith?"

They were terrified and asked each other, "Who is this? Even the wind and the waves obey him!"

They went across the lake to the region of the Gerasenes. When Jesus got out of the boat, a man with an impure spirit came from the tombs to meet him. This man lived in the tombs, and no one could bind him anymore, not even with a chain. For he had often been chained hand and foot, but he tore the chains apart and broke the irons on his feet. No one was strong enough to subdue him. Night and day among the tombs and in the hill's he would cry out and cut himself with stones.

When he saw Jesus from a distance, he ran and fell on his knees in front of him. He shouted at the top of his voice, "What do you want with me, Jesus, Son of the Most High God? In God's name don't torture me!" For Jesus had said to him, "Come out of this man, you impure spirit!"

Then Jesus asked him, "What is your name?"

"My name is Legion," he replied, "for we are many." And he begged Jesus again and again not to send them out of the area.

A large herd of pigs was feeding on the nearby hillside. The demons begged Jesus, "Send us among the pigs; allow us to go into them." He gave them permission, and the impure spirits came out and went into the pigs. The herd, about two thousand in number, rushed down the steep bank into the lake and were drowned.

Those tending the pigs ran off and reported this in the town and countryside, and the people went out to see what had happened. When they came to Jesus, they saw the man who had been possessed by the legion of demons, sitting there, dressed and in his right mind; and they were afraid. Those who had seen it told the people what had happened to the demon-possessed man—and told about the pigs as well. Then the people began to plead with Jesus to leave their region.

As Jesus was getting into the boat, the man who had been demon-possessed begged to go with him. Jesus did not let him, but said, "Go home to your own people and tell them how much the Lord has done for you, and how he has had mercy on you." So the man went away and began to tell in the Decapolis how much Jesus had done for him. And all the people were amazed.

—MARK 4:35–5:20

At first reading it is natural to think that this passage of Scripture is about the disciples and their fear of the squall wreaking havoc on their boat. I don't know about you, but I find comfort in knowing I am not the only one whose first reaction is to worry and panic in the midst of a storm. However, if we look deeper, we see this is really about the fact that the storm was a distraction to the breakthrough. The breakthrough was on the shore. Satan wanted the disciples to focus only on the storm they could see. Jesus wanted them to see the storm was merely the distraction from the miracle waiting for them on the shore.

There is always more going on in a situation than meets the natural eye. The truth is that as Christians and children of God we can walk with Jesus on a daily basis just as the disciples did. Shouldn't we be doing that? Shouldn't we talk with Him on a daily basis too? Shouldn't we experience His power, might, love, grace, and freedom on a daily basis? If that is the gift that God has given us, then why is our natural, fleshly reaction to the storms to be fearful and to panic? When our boat gets rocked a little bit, our first response is usually to cry out in fear. Here is what you need to know. Jesus was in the boat! His presence is the peace in our boat. "Now may the Lord of peace himself give you peace at all times and in every way. The Lord be with all of you" (2 Thess. 3:16).

When we are in our storms, why do we panic and act as if we have to awaken Jesus in order to be rescued and saved? Just like the disciples we proclaim, "Don't You care if we perish?" Yet all the while Jesus is in the boat! Maybe His rest and slumber were signs of what we should do when we know Jesus is in our boat. Maybe He was showing us how to react to the storm. He hasn't changed! Jesus hasn't changed! He told the disciples they were going to the other side. The storm did not catch Jesus off guard. He did not change His mind. He was going to the other side regardless of what storms arose.

SPEAK PEACE TO THE STORM

I love Jesus' response to the storm because it shows us how to respond to our storms. Let's take a closer look. First, Jesus got up! We must stop lying down and giving up in our storms and just stand up. How do we do that? Not by being spiritual streakers, running naked with only the helmet of salvation on our heads. We need to put on the full armor of God from Ephesians 6:13–17.

Second, Jesus confronted the storm. It's time to stop running from your storm and stand and confront it with the authority placed inside of you by the Holy Spirit. God's breath carries authority, and His breath flows through you! Jesus said to the storm, "Quiet! Be still!" (Mark 4:39). Next time you are in a storm, speak the Word of God over your storm. When Jesus spoke to the storm, it calmed and obeyed Him because it recognized His authority. Every storm must bow to the spoken Word of God, including the Word you speak.

Third, Jesus confronted the disciples' lack of faith and trust saying, "Why are you afraid? Do you still have no faith?" (Mark 4:40). This seems an odd question because isn't it normal to be afraid in a storm? He asked them that question because He knew they had forgotten who was in the boat. Don't forget who is in your boat! Don't forget who has authority over your storm! The Word of God— His very breath—gives you authority over the storms. Even in the midst of chaos, turmoil, fear, and disaster, there is a place called peace! It is a place where we can reside and know that Jesus is in our boat.

There is something even bigger in Jesus' rebuke of the storm that He wants us to see. He wants us to know His breath brings righteousness, peace, and joy. "The kingdom of God is…righteousness, peace and joy in the Holy Spirit [breath]" (Rom. 14:17). Jesus declared peace and calm not just to the storm but to the disciples as well. The storm was a distraction from the God's purpose in reaching the other side. There was a supernatural miracle waiting for the disciples on the other side that would birth faith in all who witnessed it. Your breakthrough over fear will spark faith in all who witness your freedom. The breath of God not only spoke to the raging storm the disciples were experiencing, but it also busted through the atmosphere and traveled all the way across the turbulent waters and reached the shore! You may not be able to see the shore because you are too frightened by the storm. Know this: your victory is on the other side of the storm. The roar the enemy is afraid of is the roar God placed inside of you to speak to the storm. Your storm must respond to the roar of the Spirit inside of you. God is speaking to you to rise up, stand, and roar His Word!

There was a demon-possessed man on the other side of the storm who needed freedom. He had no righteousness, no peace, and no joy. This man lived in inner turmoil and chaos day and night, night and day. Jesus wanted to demonstrate that His very presence brings order and unity in our lives. When He spoke peace, it caused a chain reaction that demanded a response. Not only did the elements of nature come into submission to the voice that created it, but also freedom was in progress on the shore on the other side. You see, our response to the fear of the storm will determine what happens on the other side. Jesus not only spoke to the fear of the storm but also to the aftermath of the storm. Sometimes we get so focused on the storm that we forget that there will be an aftermath to that storm.

After your storm clears, there will be debris that needs to be cleared away. What will the aftermath of your fear be? Will it be one of victory or lost breakthrough? Your miracle and deliverance is on the other side, on the shore. Don't get hung up in the storm. It is merely a distraction to delay your miracle and your breakthrough. Push through the storm and the fear and declare God's Word as you allow Him to speak to the storm. His voice gives you the authority you need over the fear. Jesus said, "Behold, I have given you authority to tread on serpents and scorpions, and over all the power of the enemy, and nothing shall hurt you" (Luke 10:19, ESV). That authority will allow you to step on the very thing the enemy tried to frighten you with. As Romans 16:20 proclaims, "The God of peace will soon crush Satan under your feet. The grace of our Lord Jesus be with you."

Jesus' voice declaring peace caused the storm in the demon-possessed man's life to submit and fall at Jesus' feet. Are you seeing this? Jesus' very voice (breath) in the storm stirred up a desire for righteousness in the man, which in return brought peace and joy. We know this because when the people came out to meet the man, he was sitting dressed and in his right mind (peace). Jesus told the man to share what had happened with his family so they would be restored (joy). While storms are indeed inevitable and circumstances are at times out of our control, we can walk in peace and joy at all times when we understand the power of Jesus' being in our boat and when we let Him speak to the storm. Seek first God's kingdom, pursue Him, and listen for His voice, and righteousness, peace, and joy will be your constant companions.

Peace is not an emotion. Peace is a place in Jesus where our spirits choose to reside. On the boat that day, Jesus was speaking peace to the very spirit of man. He said, "Peace I leave with you; my peace I give you. I do not give to you as the world gives. Do not let your hearts be troubled and do *not* be afraid" (John 14:27, emphasis added). Are you walking through a storm today? Jesus is in the storm with you. Allow God's breath to speak to your spirit and into your storm and push you to the shore to see your miracle.

Don't let the distraction called fear blind you to the breakthrough waiting on the other side of the storm. Instead declare, "Peace, be still!" Worship where you should have died! Fix your eyes on Jesus, not the storm. The prophet declared, "You will keep in perfect peace all who trust in you, all whose thoughts are fixed on you!" (Isa. 26:3, NLT). The storms are not the problem. The storms are a distraction, but they can stir us to respond and activate our faith and trust in almighty God so we might experience peace and joy like never before. Our response to the fear in the storm needs to change, and as a result of that change the aftermath will be one that brings freedom.

What happens when you finally listen for God to speak to your fear in the storm? "You will go out in joy and be led forth in peace; the mountains and hills will burst into song before you, and all the trees of the field will clap their hands" (Isa. 55:12). Not only can peace be found where fear causes a squall to arise, but also you can truly walk out joy and dance in the thunderstorm as your peace leads others to walk in peace and freedom as well. Don't let fear keep you from reaching those who need the breakthrough God has given you. Your freedom gives others permission to be free too!

The disciples experienced a storm as a means to hinder the miracle waiting on the shore of breakthrough. The storm wasn't about them. The storm was about someone on the shore who needed a miracle and freedom. The storm you are in may not be about you at all. That demon-possessed man, when faced with the very voice that broke through the storm, became one of the greatest evangelists of all time because his story speaks to everyone who reads the Word of God! If we get caught up thinking our storm is all about us, we will live in fear and never reach the shore. It's on the shore of breakthrough where you will bring hope to others who need to see you make it. Fear in the storm causes us to become very narcissistic in our walk with God. We begin to think everything is about merely surviving when God wants us to be rescuers in our breakthrough. Pat says, "Narcissism is the greatest enemy of the anointing that is on your life. The secret place has the ability to work that out of each of us. It's in the secret place that you have to look upon His face and not your own reflection in the mirror."

Are you in a storm of fear today? Are you in desperate

search of peace? If your answer is yes and you're not hearing God's voice, perhaps it is time to change your response to Him. Change how you respond to the storm and the fear. Our response is simple. We come to Him and listen and receive His gift of peace! I love the blessing in Numbers 6:24–26: "The LORD bless you and keep you; the LORD make his face shine on you and be gracious to you; the LORD turn his face toward you and give you peace." I know this to be true because a cancer diagnosis sent a storm of fear that rocked my boat to the point I felt as though I might be drowned at sea…but God! I cried out, and God heard my cry. He delivered me and spoke peace to my storm.

When I started listening for His voice above the crashing noise of the waves, I reached the shore safely. I am learning my storms are not just about me. Storms are about other people who are waiting for me and you to get to the shore to hear about our breakthrough so they will have courage arise to receive their breakthrough. Will you bring courage to others today? Take your eyes off the storm and tune your ear to hear the word "Peace" from the One who is peace—Jesus.

God's request is simple. No strings attached, no unrealistic expectations, no *thees* or *thous*. Just come! And when you come, watch as your response to come to Him changes you. Watch as your response transforms your life. In the midst of your storm stand up, wake up, confront the storm, receive peace, and embrace the obstacle as the way to the breakthrough! Then be hope to others so they too can walk in peace. If you are trying frantically to get the water out of the boat in your fear storm, turn your ears to God and hear Him speak as He beckons to your spirit, "Come and talk with Me." Will your heart's response be, "Lord, I am coming"? (See Psalm 27:8.) Don't worry about whether you feel worthy or good enough. Don't worry about what you will say. That will all get sorted out in the conversation. He simply calls to you, "Come and talk with Me." How will you respond?

CHAPTER 8

LET YOUR PRAISE BE LOUDER THAN YOUR FEAR

I bless GOD every chance I get; my lungs expand
with his praise. I live and breathe GOD; if things
aren't going well, hear this and be happy: join me in
spreading the news; together let's get the word out.

—PSALM 34:1–3, MSG

PAT AND I were at the doctor's office again, this time
for a bone marrow biopsy to help doctors determine
the extent of leukemia in my body. Our old nemesis, fear,
was trying once again to gain a foothold. The technician
drew blood before escorting us into the biopsy room to
wait for the procedure to begin. It seemed like an eternity
before the doctor came in. When he finally entered the
room, his demeanor was not at all what we expected from
someone who was about to biopsy a cancer patient.

With obvious joy he said, "Karen, I have never been
happier to walk into a patient's room and say, 'Your
blood is completely within normal range.'" Pat and I were
beyond overjoyed and stunned all at the same time. It was

a surreal moment. God had healed me—exactly what He said He would do, and yet we were shocked, momentarily disbelieving what had happened. Why do we tend to be surprised when God does what He said He will do?

Because there was no trace of the cancer, there was no reason to do a biopsy. The doctor had no explanation for the change in my blood results. "This doesn't just happen," he said. "I don't understand. It must be an aberration." *Aberration*! There was that word again! It was the very word God used when He spoke to me about fear—that fear is a learned or perceived aberration that grows into an absolute. How amazing is our Father God that He would have the doctor use that exact same word to describe my blood results?

Pat and I headed out with instructions to follow up every three months, a protocol that goes against the normal course and progression of this particular cancer. The doctor simply wanted to keep an eye on me and document my case. That day was the first time we actually used the word *cancer*. We had refused to claim it. It did not belong to us, so now we could use the word without owning it.

THE KEYS TO THE KINGDOM

The Bible promises us that God will give us the keys to the kingdom: "I will give you the keys of the kingdom of heaven; whatever you bind on earth will be bound in heaven, and whatever you loose on earth will be loosed in heaven" (Matt. 16:19). Indeed, we have seen this to be true in our own lives. God has always given us every weapon we needed to defeat

Satan's voice during our times of trial. Let me (Pat) share with you a key, a weapon that changed my life.

In the early years of our marriage Karen and I faced difficult times the way any couple does. There were times when we felt discouraged and defeated, until the Lord showed me how to counter negative thoughts from the enemy. "Just try bragging on Me a little bit, Pat, regardless of your circumstances," He said. "Then watch what happens." I hung on to that word from the Lord. When we entered the season of Karen's cancer diagnosis, we decided we would praise God—brag on Him—regardless of the circumstances. When you make up your mind to always praise God through the storm and you brag louder than Satan lies, you will be able to stand firm on God's promises in the midst of whatever is coming against you.

The enemy's number one objective is to keep us from becoming victorious. As long as we remain victims, he has us. If the devil can keep us from realizing Christ calls us and equips us to be overcomers, we will never become overcomers. That is why Peter advised believers to "be alert and of sober mind. Your enemy the devil prowls around like a roaring lion looking for someone to devour" (1 Pet. 5:8). Did you catch that? It says the enemy is like a lion. Satan tries to act like a lion, but he is never a lion. He's nothing more than a copycat. We know Jesus is our true Lion, the Lion of the tribe of Judah! Proverbs 30:30 characterizes the Lion of Judah perfectly: "the lion, which is mightiest among beasts and does not turn back before any" (esv). That's right! Jesus is *the* mighty victor, and He doesn't turn back—ever!

Satan is such a liar. His number one job is to deceive us

with lies. Jesus gave us the devil's résumé in John 8:44: "He was a murderer from the beginning, not holding to the truth, for there is no truth in him. When he lies, he speaks his native language, for he is a liar and the father of lies." In fact, his very title, devil (Greek *diabolos*), means "accusing falsely…false accuser, slanderer."[1] It has been my experience that every time God gets ready to use someone for His kingdom purposes, the first thing he must do is conquer the irrational voices seeking to silence the vision at hand. There comes a moment when you must quiet the voices of fear and defeat by being louder and more boisterous in your praise!

For years the voice of the enemy held me hostage. Why? Because he knew that if I ever got past his lies, I would step into my destiny. You see, not only is he a liar, but the Bible also declares Satan is "the accuser of our brethren" (Rev. 12:10, NKJV). The word *accuser* in Revelation 12:10 is *katēgoreō* in the Greek, which means to accuse or make an accusation before a judge.[2] One of its synonyms means "to make verbal assault which reaches its goal."[3]

The very nature of Satan is to whisper threats and demeaning accusations against the saints of God. The devil will lie to you about who you are and accuse you of being what you are not, with the goal of intimidating you until you become afraid. As believers we all must watch out for him at all times. We must learn to distinguish the voice of God from the whispers or shouts of defeat. We are not only called to overcome but to shout louder than our doubt, because the power of bragging on God changes everything.

For though we live in the world, we do not wage war as the world does. The weapons we fight with are not the weapons of the world. On the contrary, they have divine power to demolish strongholds. We demolish arguments and every pretension that sets itself up against the knowledge of God, and we take captive every thought to make it obedient to Christ.

—2 CORINTHIANS 10:3–5

BRAG ON GOD

Let me share a little about the day God spoke to me about the power of bragging on Him. I'll never forget it. It was September 2015, and I was in a hotel in Phoenix, scheduled to speak at a church conference later that day. Very early in the morning I was awakened by the Holy Spirit. Suddenly I heard the Lord say to me, "Pat, have you ever noticed that when I do miracles in a service, they happen when you talk about what I am doing instead of what you are doing?"

"Lord," I replied, "what do you mean? I always share of Your goodness."

"Son, I am looking for those who will do more than just share about Me," God said. "I'm looking for those who will brag on Me, those who will declare My goodness in the land. There's a difference."

Those words got me out of bed. Immediately I arose and began to write a message about bragging on God. Over time I realized that when I practice bragging on God, there is no room for the enemy to place fear or insecurity in my life. You see, when you brag on God, it restores your spirit man and quiets the voice of the enemy. When you brag on God, His presence overwhelms every situation. This is because He is our "right now" God. Right now the angels in heaven are declaring, "Holy, holy, holy," not, "Maybe, maybe, maybe." God is always on the throne, worthy of all praise, as He continually makes all things new (Rev. 21:5). Only He can restart your life. He is a restorer of the lost and the refresher of the weary. He is God, and He never abandons His post. He does not leave us to fend for ourselves. He is always worthy of our constant praise. Even as I write this chapter, an overwhelming excitement fills my soul, leading me to that place of praise!

PRAISE BREAK

Sing to GOD, everyone and everything! Get out his salvation news every day! Publish his glory among the godless nations, his wonders to all races and religions. And why? Because GOD is great—well worth praising! No god or goddess comes close in honor. All the popular gods are stuff and nonsense, but GOD made the cosmos! Splendor and majesty flow out of him, strength and joy fill his place. Shout Bravo! to GOD, families of the peoples, in awe of the Glory, in awe of the Strength: Bravo! Shout Bravo! to his famous Name, lift high an offering and enter his presence!

Stand resplendent in his robes of holiness! God is serious business, take him seriously; he's put the earth in place and it's not moving. So let Heaven rejoice, let Earth be jubilant, and pass the word among the nations, "GOD reigns!" Let Ocean, all teeming with life, bellow, let Field and all its creatures shake the rafters; then the trees in the forest will add their applause to all who are pleased and present before GOD—he's on his way to set things right!

—1 CHRONICLES 16:23–31, MSG

I'm thanking you, GOD, from a full heart, I'm writing the book on your wonders. I'm whistling, laughing, and jumping for joy; I'm singing your song, High God.

—PSALM 9:1–2, MSG

As you read the remainder of this chapter, you'll find several praise breaks. Stop and take a moment to brag on God, and let your praise be your weapon.

BEHOLD HIM AGAIN

Have you noticed that so many worship songs and sermons today are about us and not God? Maybe this is why we see very few miracles. Somewhere along the way the gospel message became about how great we can be instead of how great our God already is. If we are not careful, our church services will be built around reminding one another who we are instead of who He is! I think we often don't want to hear who God is for fear of forgetting who we are. The fact is that if we will stay at the cross, we will realize Jesus is the center of it all. It was the cross that allowed us to experience the 2 Corinthians 5:17 life: "Therefore, if anyone is in Christ, the new creation has come: The old has gone, the new is here!"

We change when we behold Him because you will become what you behold. Beholding Him means our lives should be different as we are "transformed into his image with ever-increasing glory" (2 Cor. 3:18). If you will look on the goodness of God, it will change your posture toward Him. Instead of fear and dread, you will be filled with awe and excitement. It is about sitting at His feet once again as a child with expectancy. Look what Romans 8:15–17 says in *The Message* paraphrase:

> This resurrection life you received from God is not a timid, grave-tending life. It's adventurously expectant, greeting God with a childlike "What's next, Papa?" God's Spirit touches our spirits and confirms who we really are. We know who He is, and we know who we are: Father and children. And we know we are going to get what's coming to us—an unbelievable inheritance! We go through exactly what Christ goes through. If we go through the hard times with him, then we're certainly going to go through the good times with him!

Did you catch that? You get to say, "What's next, Papa?" I truly believe that at His feet we regain our footing. When there is less of my issue and more of His glory, then suddenly the scenery changes! The equation changes to "no more of me" because I stand in awe of the fact that God always has time for me.

GOD IS USING THE BRAGGERS

I believe God is not looking for the most talented or gifted. He isn't looking for the most brilliant or even those connected to the right people. God is looking for those who are available. First Corinthians 1 describes whom God uses.

PRAISE BREAK

God is the awesome, majestic, mighty, all-powerful, all-encompassing, all-knowing, all-seeing, compassionate, supernatural, all-loving, fiercely jealous, without excuse, mind-altering, heart-rendering, soul-purchasing, spirit-reviving, bondage-breaking, peace-empowering, covenant-creating, Satan-crushing, bride-washing, dominion-releasing I Am Who I Am!

Heaven is His throne, and earth is His footstool (Isa. 66:1).

Praise the LORD, my soul; all my inmost being, praise his holy name. Praise the LORD, my soul, and forget not all his benefits—who forgives all your sins and heals all your diseases, who redeems your life from the pit and crowns you with love and compassion, who satisfies your desires with good things so that your youth is renewed like the eagle's. The LORD works righteousness and justice for all the oppressed.

—PSALM 103:1–6

Take a good look, friends, at who you were when you got called into this life. I don't see many of "the brightest and the best" among you, not many influential, not many from high-society families. Isn't it obvious that God deliberately chose men and women that the culture overlooks and exploits and abuses, chose these "nobodies" to expose the hollow pretensions of the "somebodies"?

—1 CORINTHIANS 1:26–28, MSG

These are the kingdom shakers who do not need accolades or large numbers of followers on social media. Why does God use these people? All you have to do is the read the next three verses—"so that no one may boast before him. It is because of him that you are in Christ Jesus, who has become for us wisdom from God—that is, our righteousness, holiness and redemption. Therefore, as it is written: 'Let the one who boasts boast in the Lord'" (1 Cor. 1:29–31). When you brag on God, it suddenly replaces your flesh man with a spirit man who has been dying to get out! Let's look more closely at the characteristics of braggers from Scripture.

> They realize they did not get where they are on their own: "We thank you, God, we thank you—your Name is our favorite word; your mighty works are all we talk about" (Ps. 75:1, MSG).

> They realize if God uses them, then He gets all of the praise: "If anyone speaks, they should do so as one who speaks the very words of God. If anyone serves, they should do so with the strength God provides, so that in all things God may be praised through Jesus Christ. To him be the glory and the power for ever and ever. Amen" (1 Pet. 4:11).

> They are fearless: "Pray also for me, that whenever I speak, words may be given me so that I will fearlessly make known the mystery of the gospel, for which I am an ambassador in chains. Pray that I may declare it fearlessly, as I should" (Eph. 6:19–20).

> They have abandoned the mirror of self-deprecation to once again look out the window of harvest: "But as for me, it is good to be near God. I have

made the Sovereign Lord my refuge; I will tell of all your deeds" (Ps. 73:28).

Somewhere along the way they realized that without God they are nothing: "But he said to me, 'My grace is sufficient for you, for my power is made perfect in weakness.' Therefore, I will boast all the more gladly about my weaknesses, so that Christ's power may rest on me. That is why, for Christ's sake, I delight in weaknesses, in insults, in hardships, in persecutions, in difficulties. For when I am weak, then I am strong" (2 Cor. 12:9–10).

They realize that if they will just lift Jesus up, then He will do the rest: "Now is the time for judgment on this world; now the prince of this world will be driven out. And I, when I am lifted up from the earth, will draw all people to myself" (John 12:31–32).

PRAISE BREAK

Praise the Lord. Praise God in his sanctuary; praise him in his mighty heavens. Praise him for his acts of power; praise him for his surpassing greatness. Praise him with the sounding of the trumpet, praise him with the harp and lyre, praise him with timbrel and dancing, praise him with the strings and pipe, praise him with the clash of cymbals, praise him with resounding cymbals. Let everything that has breath praise the Lord. Praise the Lord.

—Psalm 150

They understand where their strength comes from: "But you, dear friends, by building yourselves up in your most holy faith and praying in the Holy Spirit, keep yourselves in God's love as you wait for the mercy of our Lord Jesus Christ to bring you to eternal life" (Jude 20–21).

The days ahead will require a new level of praise. We must keep our eyes on Jesus, who both began and finished this race we are in. The Scripture tells us: "Keep your eyes on Jesus, who both began and finished this race we're in. Study how he did it. Because he never lost sight of where he was headed—that exhilarating finish in and with God—he could put up with anything along the way: Cross, shame, whatever. And now he's there, in the place of honor, right alongside God" (Heb. 12:2–3, MSG).

Be assured that as you run your race, culture will challenge you at every level. If you believe in biblical truth, you will be found guilty in the court of public opinion. This will take place when relative truth is challenged by God's absolute truth. We are living in a time when right is wrong and wrong is right, with the forces of political correctness and cognitive dissonance fighting for our minds. That is why we must learn to praise regardless of what happens to us. As the apostle Peter did, I implore you to keep praising. "Dear friends, do not be surprised at the fiery ordeal that has come on you to test you, as though something strange were happening to you. But rejoice inasmuch as you participate in the sufferings of Christ, so that you may be overjoyed when his glory is revealed" (1 Pet. 4:12–13).

PRAISE BREAK

Arise, shine, for your light has come, and the glory of the LORD rises upon you. See, darkness covers the earth and thick darkness is over the peoples, but the LORD rises upon you and his glory appears over you. Nations will come to your light, and kings to the brightness of your dawn. Lift up your eyes and look about you: All assemble and come to you; your sons come from afar, and your daughters are carried on the hip. Then you will look and be radiant, your heart will throb and swell with joy; the wealth on the seas will be brought to you, to you the riches of the nations will come.

—ISAIAH 60:1–5

THE FOURTH MAN IS IN THE FIRE

There are so many amazing stories in God's Word that prove if you praise Him, God will handle whatever situation is trying to destroy you. Whether it was Moses versus Pharaoh, David versus Goliath, or Paul and Silas in prison, our God always showed up as a great defender. One story in this regard took place during the days of Babylonian captivity. There was an evil king named Nebuchadnezzar, who ruled the Babylonian empire. He conquered nation after nation, including Judah (Dan. 1:1). As he conquered each nation, he forced the best minds, the best warriors, and the most talented to become slaves in his administration. Among those enslaved were Daniel, Shadrach, Meshach, and Abednego (Dan. 1:6–7). "To these four young men God gave knowledge and understanding of all kinds of literature and learning. And Daniel could understand visions and dreams of all kinds" (Dan. 1:17). God gave them favor and then raised them up in the king's administration (Dan. 2:48–49). I have found that God always raises up a remnant at the darkest of times. They are the ones who will stand when others will not.

Nebuchadnezzar also raided and stole all of the articles found in the temples and places of worship in the nations he conquered. He then placed the articles in his demonic temple of Baal (Dan. 1:2) in the hope that maybe one of the gods and idols would have power. He made sacrifices to the idols, yet nothing happened. Finally, he decided to build an idol himself.

> King Nebuchadnezzar made an image of gold, sixty cubits high and six cubits wide, and set it up on the plain of Dura in the province of Babylon.... Then the herald loudly proclaimed, "Nations and peoples of every language, this is what you are commanded to do: As soon as you hear the sound of the horn, flute, zither, lyre, harp, pipe and all kinds of music, you must fall down and worship the image of gold that King Nebuchadnezzar has set up. Whoever does not fall down and worship will immediately be thrown into a blazing furnace."
>
> —DANIEL 3:1, 4–6

Then the challenge came! Word got back to the king that three Jewish officials—Shadrach, Meshach, and Abednego—refused to bow. Nebuchadnezzar had them brought before him and told them to either bow or face the fiery furnace. As you know from Scripture, they refused to bow. In fact they said to the king, "If we are thrown into the blazing furnace, the God we serve is able to deliver us from it, and he will deliver us from Your Majesty's hand" (Dan. 3:17).

The next verse is amazing: "But even if he does not, we want you to know, Your Majesty, that we will not serve your gods or worship the image of gold you have set up" (Dan. 3:18). That is what I call a "but if not" praise. A "but if not" praise is when you have made up your mind that if even God never does anything else for you, what He has already done is enough to warrant your praise.

The king was so mad that he ordered the furnace to be heated seven times hotter. Shadrach, Meshach, and Abednego were then thrown into the fire. That was when God decided to join them in the furnace. Suddenly Nebuchadnezzar realized that not only were the three men not burning, but there was a fourth man in the fire: "Look! I see four men walking around in the fire, unbound and unharmed, and the fourth looks like a son of the gods" (Dan. 3:25). Wow! He was seeing Jesus in the fire with them. When they were brought out, there was not a burn mark on them! In fact watch as God drops the mic!

> Nebuchadnezzar said, "Blessed be the God of Shadrach, Meshach, and Abednego! He sent his angel and rescued his servants who trusted in him! They ignored the king's orders and laid their bodies on the line rather than serve or worship any god but their own. Therefore I issue

this decree: Anyone anywhere, of any race, color, or creed, who says anything against the God of Shadrach, Meshach, and Abednego will be ripped to pieces, limb from limb, and their houses torn down. There has never been a god who can pull off a rescue like this." Then the king promoted Shadrach, Meshach, and Abednego in the province of Babylon.

—DANIEL 3:28–30, MSG

RELEASE YOUR ROAR!

If you will stand firm, have faith, and praise God regardless of what you are going through, God will reward you. He says so right in His Word: "And without faith it is impossible to please God, because anyone who comes to him must believe that he exists and that he rewards those who earnestly seek him" (Heb. 11:6). Now, let me tell you more about the fourth man so the next time fear tries to overwhelm you, you can stand firm and release your roar with bragging words that come straight from the Word of God![4]

In Genesis Jesus is the seed of the woman.

In Exodus He is the Passover Lamb.

In Leviticus He is the High Priest.

In Numbers He is the pillar of cloud by day and the pillar of fire by night.

In Deuteronomy He is the Prophet like unto Moses.

In Joshua He is the commander of the Lord's army.

In Judges He is the judge and lawgiver.

In Ruth He is the kinsman-redeemer.

In 1 and 2 Samuel He is the stone of help.

In Kings and Chronicles He is the reigning King.

In Ezra He is the faithful scribe.

In Nehemiah He is the rebuilder of the broken-down walls of human life.

In Esther He is our Mordecai.

In Job He is the ever-living Redeemer.

In Psalms He is the rock.

In Proverbs and Ecclesiastes He is wisdom.

In the Song of Solomon He is the lover and the Bridegroom.

In Isaiah He is the Prince of Peace.

In Jeremiah He is the righteous Branch.

In Lamentations He is our portion.

In Ezekiel He is the watchman.

In Daniel He is the fourth man in the fiery furnace.

In Hosea He is the faithful husband, forever married to the backslider.

In Joel He is the baptizer with the Holy Ghost.

In Amos He is the burden bearer.

In Obadiah He is the Deliverer.

In Jonah He is the great missionary.

In Micah He is the One who casts our sin into the sea.

In Nahum He is the messenger who brings good tidings and peace.

In Habakkuk He is God's evangelist, crying, "Revive thy work in the midst of the years" (3:2, KJV).

In Zephaniah He is the Savior.

In Haggai He is the restorer of lost heritage.

In Zechariah He is the fountain opened for the house of David for sin and uncleanness.

In Malachi He is the sun of righteousness, rising with healing in His wings.

In Matthew He is the Son of God.

In Mark He is the miracle worker.

In Luke He is the Son of Man.

In John He is the Messiah.

In Acts He is the Holy Spirit.

In Romans He is our justifier.

In Corinthians He is the gifts of the Spirit.

In Galatians He is the liberty by which we stand.

In Ephesians He is the unsearchable riches.

In Philippians He is the God who supplies all our needs.

In Colossians He is the fullness of the Godhead bodily.

In 1 and 2 Thessalonians He is the Comforter.

In 1 and 2 Timothy He is the ransom for all.

In Titus He is the blessed hope.

In Philemon He is the Mediator.

In Hebrews He is the author and finisher of our faith.

In James He is the great physician.

In 1 and 2 Peter He is the Chief Shepherd.

In 1, 2, and 3 John He is everlasting love.

In Jude He is the Lord coming with ten thousand of His saints.

In Revelation He is the Alpha and the Omega, the first and the last, the beginning and the end, the King of kings, and the Lord of lords.

Jesus is:

Adonai Jehovah—Lord God, or Sovereign Lord

El Elyon—the Most High God

El Olam—the everlasting God

El Shaddai—the almighty God

Jehovah Eloheenu—the Lord our God

Jehovah Elohim—the Lord God

Jehovah Hoseenu—the Lord our Maker

Jehovah Jireh—the Lord our Provider

Jehovah Mekoddishkem—the Lord our Sanctifier

Jehovah Nissi—the Lord my Banner

Jehovah Rohi—the Lord my Shepherd

Jehovah Ropheka—the Lord your Healer

Jehovah Sabaoth—the Lord of Hosts

Jehovah Shalom—the Lord is peace

Jehovah Shammah—the Lord is there

Jehovah Tsidkenu—the Lord our Righteousness

CHAPTER 9

THE HIDDEN

For no matter where I am, even when I'm far from
home, I will cry out to you for a father's help. When
I'm feeble and overwhelmed by life, guide me
into your glory, where I am safe and sheltered.

—PSALM 61:2, TPT

RUNNING AND HIDING has always been a natural reaction to fear. As a result fear has the ability to cause us to withdraw and go into seclusion. This is called self-preservation. Even as children, when we were in trouble, nearly all of us ran and hid for fear of the consequences about to come down on us. This response to fear is not new. It has gone on since the creation and fall of man. Adam and Eve never experienced fear until they took a bite from the fruit of the tree of the knowledge of good and evil. At that moment, the sinful nature took over and what did they do? They ran and hid.

When God strode through the garden, He looked for Adam. But Adam and Eve heard God coming, and realizing the ultimate evil they had committed, they hid behind the trees. God found them and asked them why they were hiding. Do you know what Adam said? He said, "I heard Your voice in the garden and was afraid because I was naked, so I hid myself" (Gen. 3:10, MEV). Man may have hidden *from* God in the garden, but in Christ, God has called us to hide *in* Him. He is always ready to whisk us away so He can secure His greatest creation, you and me: "For he will conceal me there when troubles come; he will hide me in his sanctuary. He will place me out of reach on a high rock" (Ps. 27:5, NLT).

We must realize that even though fear may cause us to hide, it does not mean God is not with us. God is always with us. The psalmist proclaimed, "Lord, even when your path takes me through the valley of deepest darkness, fear will never conquer me, for you already have! You remain close to me and lead me through it all the way. Your authority is my strength and my peace. The comfort of your love takes away my fear. I'll never be lonely, for you are near" (Ps. 23:4, TPT). Fear can actually be the vehicle God uses to transform us. God will use your season of hiding to transform you and grow you into who He originally designed you to be. God always takes what was meant for bad and uses it to restore His original plan. He will use your season of hiding to teach you, cultivate you, discipline you, and even equip you.

Jesus said, "For nothing is hidden, except to be revealed; nor has anything been secret, but that it would come to light" (Mark 4:22, NASB). He certainly understood this truth. Just look at the Gospels and you will see that Jesus spent most of His life in hiding. Even when in the fullness of time God revealed Jesus to the world, He "often withdrew to lonely places and prayed" (Luke 5:16). Jesus would disappear to spend time alone with the Father because He understood it was in solitude that He could best hear His Father speak. What does that tell us? It tells us that when fear strikes, it is not time to run away from God and hide but time to run and hide *with* God the Father. Regardless of what forced you into hiding, use that time to meet once again with God. This is a biblical principle illustrated throughout Scripture.

- Out of fear Moses' mother hid him in a river when he was a baby. Then later Moses was afraid and hid in the desert from his past, but God used that season to kill all of the old in him and prepare him for greatness.

- Gideon was afraid and hiding in a winepress when God told him that he would raise him up.

- David, as a shepherd in the fields, was hidden as he killed the lion and the bear. He was even hidden from Samuel when he first appeared and had to be brought in from the field. First Samuel 16:7 says, "But the LORD said to Samuel, 'Do not consider his appearance or his height, for I have rejected him. The LORD does not look at the things people look at. People look at the

> outward appearance, but the LORD looks at the heart.'"

- When the apostle Paul first found Christ, he was forced to disappear for three years because of the fear caused by his past actions, until such time as his message could be received by the church. The one who brought fear would be used to bring hope to the world because Jesus redeemed him.

- John the Revelator was exiled to the island of Patmos, but God allowed him to experience heaven while living alone on a deserted island.

I (Pat) have said for years, "The greater the anointing, the greater the isolation." I know what it is to feel hidden, to feel alone, to feel put on the shelf in the wilderness. So many know Karen as a powerful preacher and author. Yet they do not know that for years Karen desired to be used by God, but she had dealt with shyness her entire life. I can remember asking her to share in the early years of ministry, and she would literally break out in hives. Then one day something shifted in her. She suddenly conquered her fear and decided now was the time. She didn't realize God had waited for the right time for her to arise and proclaim His Word boldly. Her season of shyness was actually God cultivating a fire deep within. Now her message is heard literally around the world, but first it had to be heard in her prayer closet where she spent time talking to God.

Are you feeling that way? I think many experience seasons

of hiding. Be encouraged! I feel in my spirit that God will take your hidden seasons and use them to make you His big reveal! Fear may have sent you into hiding, but your burden to heal others will eventually bring you out of hiding. Here is a prophetic word the Lord gave me in that regard:

> Are you hidden? Then I have good news for you! God has His telescope to His eye! He is searching for the "hidden"! These are those who are leaving isolation to help lead His visitation. God is bypassing those who have become so entitled that they smell like greenrooms and not sheep, so narcissistic that they look past the hurting and stare at the mirror, so self-reliant that they can now avoid the secret place, so greedy for acceptance that they have chosen relevance over the reverence. You see, God always chooses the ones who have disappeared into anonymity in order to learn how ravens feed and brooks keep bubbling. The marching orders are being sent out to the forgotten. The orders are clear: Decrease, and He will increase. Catch aflame, and they will come watch you burn! Declare the hope of the cross and exalt His name. Reach the hurting, lost, and broken for they are future citizenry of heaven! "Yet even now!"

In the hidden season God does His greatest work. Use your hidden seasons to be restored in God. The psalmist said, "God is a safe place to hide, ready to help when we need him. We stand fearless at the cliff-edge of doom, courageous in seastorm and earthquake, before the rush and roar of oceans, the tremors that shift mountains. Jacob-wrestling God fights for us, GOD-of-Angel-Armies protects us" (Ps. 46:1–3, MSG). Trust His timing. The calling of God without the timing of God will result in the absence of God!

Let me share a story I wrote about in my book *Why Is God So Mad at Me?*:

> Years ago my family went through a rough season in ministry. I had moved the family and ministry to Las Vegas, Nevada, in hope of enlarging our organization. Soon after our move my wife and I realized that it was not God's plan for our life. I had missed it big-time. I have learned that *the calling of God without the timing of God results in the absence of God!* Ambition and passion got in the way of wisdom and proper planning.
>
> Despite that, our family grew closer in every aspect during that season. More importantly I grew closer to God. I became more reliant on God than I had ever been in my life. It was truly the best of times and the worst of times. It was during this season that God gave me a revelation that He wants to be our friend, not just our Savior and Lord.
>
> I was driving home from the airport one day when a song came on the radio. The singer was one of my favorite musicians, Israel Houghton, and the song began with Israel simply asking God who we humans are that He would be mindful of us and hear us when we call out to Him. Then later in the song Israel declared over and over that we are friends of God—that He calls us His friends.

Those lyrics were unbelievable to me. God called me His friend?

I had to pull over to the side of the road because this song was ministering to me so deeply. God began to speak to me and give me direction for both my family and the ministry. It was one of those powerful moments of revelation straight from heaven. That was the day I realized God truly is my friend. I realized that He cared about me, that He loved me, and that He wanted to spend time with me and give me the direction I so desperately needed.

I must have played that song a thousand times over the next few months. My heart's cry is to always be a friend of God. That's one reason I love Proverbs 22:11: ["One who loves a pure heart and who speaks with grace will have the king for a friend."] If there's one thing I know for sure, it's that I want the King to be my friend.[1]

CHRONOS TIME OR *KAIROS* TIME

We tend to only like God's timing if it is according to our time (*chronos*) instead of realizing we must wait on His timing (*kairos*). Often we believe that God has placed us in time-out, or the wilderness season, due to our lack of gifting, a circle of influence, knowledge, or even a stage persona when actually it is because He is a good Father. Good fathers protect their children from the image that culture desires to create. Philippians 1:6 says, "…being confident of this, that he who began a good work in you will carry it on to completion until the day of Christ Jesus." We must all learn to praise while in obscurity and anonymity. Why? Because each one of us is a precious possibility! We are constantly learning what it means to praise with no motive other than our passionate love for Jesus that keeps drawing us to Him. God raises up the faithful ones, those who live with burning hearts of love for the One who is love. There is an obscure story in 2 Chronicles of one woman who tried to destroy destiny.

> When Athaliah the mother of Ahaziah saw that her son was dead, she proceeded to destroy the whole royal family of the house of Judah. But Jehosheba, the daughter of King Jehoram, took Joash son of Ahaziah and stole him away from among the royal princes who were about to be murdered and put him and his nurse in a bedroom. Because Jehosheba, the daughter of King Jehoram and wife of the priest Jehoiada, was Ahaziah's sister, she hid the child from Athaliah so she could not kill him. He remained hidden with them at the temple of God for six years while Athaliah ruled the land.
>
> —2 CHRONICLES 22:10–12

Athaliah was the daughter of the evil Queen Jezebel and King Ahab. Remember, it was Jezebel who killed the prophets of God. Her daughter took her mother's evil to another level by trying to kill all of the anointed ones so none could fulfill God's call. When Athaliah found out her son was dead, she decided that she would run the kingdom. To do this, she had to kill off all the rightful heirs to the throne. Overcome with evil, she ran into the nursery where all her grandsons were and proceeded to slaughter them. As she went about her hideous task of destroying the royal seed, one brave couple, Jehosheba and Jehoiada, rescued one little boy named Joash. Rightfully fearing for Joash's life, they hid him for six years in the house of God. I believe the spirit of Athaliah is running rampant today. It is a spirit killing the next generation, taking out the newborn Christians with its number one goal being to thwart kingdom destiny.

REJOICE IN THE HIDDEN SEASON

If you feel the stirring of incompleteness—that you have been hidden for a season with dreams yet to be fulfilled—hear me out. We all want an exit door to our desert. Yet the truth is that God often does His mightiest works in secret, in our hidden seasons. I believe you have been hidden so God can separate you for *your* next! Did you catch that? Not *His* next but *your* next. God always calls His special people out of the crowd and puts them in the alone place to do something in them and through them. That is because in the kingdom equation rejection is protection. God does His greatest work in the waiting room. Karen and I have a picture in a hallway in our home. It has the words "Until God opens the next door, worship in the hallway." You see, we have decided that we are not seeking God's hands to provide or His feet to lead us but rather His face (2 Chron. 7:14) so that we learn His character. We learned a long time ago that God's timing is way better than man's favor. Our goal is to simply wait on God. Just as Habakkuk said, "This vision is for a future time.

It describes the end, and it will be fulfilled. If it seems slow in coming, wait patiently, for it will surely take place. It will not be delayed" (Hab. 2:3, NLT). Your delay is due process in action! God is preparing the way for you.

Expectant parents today have every kind of party, even gender reveal parties. Well, let me tell you that heaven is about to have an anointing reveal and the colors are not pink or blue. Heaven's revelation is gold and purple—the royal colors of God's anointing. God is about to awaken priests and kings to reveal to the world those He has chosen. Joash was hidden for six years. Six years! Yet six years of hiding led to forty years of blessing. Scripture says that "in the seventh year Jehoiada showed his strength" (2 Chron. 23:1) and crowned seven-year-old Joash king. Joash reigned for forty years. Jehoiada restored the priesthood by his action. The name Jehoiada means "Jehovah knows."[2] God knew Joash's destiny all along, hiding him for six years, until it was his time.

The Athaliah spirit is the daughter of the Jezebel spirit. It not only kills the anointing, but it also tries to make sure those with God's anointing never reach maturity. Athaliah wanted to kill the anointing, kill the house of David, kill the seeds of royalty. Yet God directed one woman to hide the precious possibility that He destined. God sometimes hides what He needs to protect until it is ready to overcome. That was true for Joash, and it could be true for you as well. Out of your hiddenness can come the greatest revelation of God's purpose for your life. What starts as fear and self-preservation can actually become the story that leads to your restoration. God has the power to change sleepers into reapers, orphans into sons and daughters, and widows into brides.

> Hear, O LORD, and be gracious to me; O LORD, be my helper. You have turned for me my mourning into dancing; You have loosed my sackcloth and girded me with gladness, that my soul may sing praise to You and not be silent. O LORD my God, I will give thanks to You forever.
> —PSALM 30:10–12, NASB

Joash was hidden so the house of David could continue. And it had to continue because it was from the house of David that Jesus Christ would come. God's big reveal was destined to come from the house of David. Romans 1:3 says, "The Good News is about his Son. In his earthly life he was born into King David's family line" (NLT). If Joash needed to be hidden for a season, then don't despair when you are in your hidden season. Nothing can thwart the will of God. Don't think God is trying to violate you in your hidden season. He is not. God will hide you to validate and vindicate you so you can step into your destiny.

Get ready to come out of hiding! God is going to use you. You are needed for this next great awakening. God has not sidelined you. He is just waiting until you are ready before He reveals you! Your hidden season is how He protects the anointing from the anointing killers. Get ready to dream again! Think of the life of Joseph. Thrown into a pit by his brothers, Joseph started his journey in fear. He went from dreamer to worker to prisoner until he became ruler. The dream had to endure the process of the hidden season until God's appointed time.

You are the hidden! You are God's precious possibility! We need you! In fact, all of creation needs you. I believe your appointed time is now, and God is ready to have a reveal party with your name on the box. The Bible says, "For the creation waits in eager expectation for the children of God to be revealed" (Rom. 8:19). Take your fear and make it the embryo of courage. We are destined to be God's ambassadors of hope. In our hidden seasons we become caches of God's hope, ordained to be "Jesus with skin on" in a hurting world. God is whispering to you even now—"What I tell you now in the darkness, shout abroad when daybreak comes. What I whisper in your ear, shout from the housetops for all to hear!" (Matt. 10:27, NLT). He is reassuring you that He will use your pain to heal others.

CHAPTER 10

DON'T GIVE UP; GET MOVING!

> Now there were four men with leprosy at the
> entrance of the city gate. They said to each other,
> "Why stay here until we die? If we say, 'We'll go
> into the city'—the famine is there, and we will die.
> And if we stay here, we will die. So let's go over to
> the camp of the Arameans and surrender. If they
> spare us, we live; if they kill us, then we die."
>
> —2 KINGS 7:3–4

HAVE YOU EVER walked through something that just made you want to give up? Does the obstacle in front of you seem impossible to overcome at times? Are there times when you feel as if even one step forward requires more strength than you can muster? If you are answering yes to any of these questions, I (Karen) am here to tell you that it is time to stop looking at the obstacle in front of you and start realizing God is in control. God is with you, and He will give you the strength and power to take one more step. If you will just take that one step, it will make all the difference in the outcome.

All of us experience times in life when we take a hit, when something happens, and we can either jump up and keep going, or we lie there and let whatever hit us overcome us. For example, there I was one day, trying to carry several items and walking backward through our condo at the beach while listening to Abby from the other room. I am so impatient that I didn't want to make multiple trips or wait for help, so I tried to do more than I could. Lo and behold, my foot slipped! In my attempt to not drop anything, I couldn't grab hold of anything to keep from falling. My hip slammed into a desk along the wall, and I fell straight back and hit my head on the opposite wall and dropped everything I was so desperately trying to hold on to. It was quite the scene, and I am so glad no one was there in the hallway to witness my horrible fall.

For a brief moment I thought about just lying there in a crumpled heap and giving in to the pain and humiliation. Fear tried to take hold of me and cause me to feel as though maybe I had broken a bone or sustained a concussion. I had just recently had a disc removed in my neck. What if I dislocated the new bone graft? Lying there afraid to move, I remembered an annoying commercial that comes on too often when we watch our favorite family TV series. It is a rude commercial that reminds us we are getting old, a body in motion stays in motion, and a body at rest stays at rest.

Thankfully that rude commercial shook me out of my fear. Knowing I needed to get back in motion, I jumped up and just shook off the fall. If I had just lain there, the pain could have gotten even worse as my muscles and joints began to swell from inflammation. Getting up right away and walking off the fall loosened up my muscles, allowing them recover. You get where I'm going with this, I'm sure. When life causes us to fall in some way, the best thing we can do in response is to get up right away and keep moving. It can be tempting to give in to pain, fear, and humiliation and just wallow in failure, but that is the wrong response. God wants us to get up and get moving and let Him fight for us.

Life will cause us to fall—that is certain. And we can also bring about our own falls just as I did that day in the condo at the beach. In an effort to grasp everything, we sometimes lose our footing and drop it all. Fear of being inadequate can cause us to take on too much. Unrealistic, self-imposed expectations can do the same. The truth is we are often inadequate, but God is always more than adequate. He doesn't expect us to do it all alone. With Him we can win. Without Him we often end up throwing our hands in the air, giving up, and staying on the floor in defeat. Today is the best day to realize you do not have to sit in defeat any longer! It's time to get up and get moving! It's time to get up out of your fear and failure and pain and get yourself back in the game.

I no longer take this life for granted. From the time I was diagnosed with cancer to the time God healed me, I was able to think about how I wanted my life to count. I had to decide whether I would I lay down and accept defeat or get up and do something. We have to fight for the things that matter most. Great accomplishments and mighty feats are not usually just handed to us on a silver platter. We have to fight for our health, our marriages, our families, and our dreams and purposes. God has great and mighty plans for us, and the enemy wants to derail those plans. Satan's goal is to intimidate you into backing into a corner in fear and defeat. The enemy will do whatever it takes to knock you down and distract you from reaching the prize at the end of your race. Satan is the bully on the school playground, and fear is his weapon. He will throw sickness at you and throw challenges and troubles at you at every turn just to get you off course. Fear always loves an audience.

It's time to say, "No more!" Determine right now that whatever the enemy throws at you will fail. Declare, "Satan, you will not take me out! I will live every day fulfilling God's plan and purpose for my life." God has given us every weapon we need to defeat the enemy along with spiritual armor to protect us. He does not leave us helpless. Satan will try to forge weapons against you. He will surround you at times. He will attack on occasion. But here is the best part, straight from Scripture—"No weapon that is formed against you will prosper" (Isa. 54:17, NASB).

KEEP GOING, AND PUSH THROUGH; GOD IS WITH YOU

I will never forget preaching in south Alabama one Sunday evening. It was in the midst of the toughest part of our battle with the cancer diagnosis. I was preaching on being undone in God's presence. I had not gotten very far into the message when a woman walked right up to the front of the altar area and just stared at me. It seemed odd, but

I thought maybe she was coming to the altar to pray. That was not her intent. She stood right in front of me and just stared at me. It appeared that no one else in the room even noticed her. I continued to preach, and as I did, she began to speak curses toward me and call me names. It was distracting to say the least; however, as she stood there, everything seemed to move slow motion. I was preaching, but I was fully aware of her trying to intimidate me.

I almost stopped preaching, wondering why no one else seemed bothered by her. All of a sudden the Holy Spirit spoke to me and said, "Karen, do not stop preaching. Do not give attention to the enemy. Just keep going and push through it." In that moment, I realized that giving up and giving in was exactly what the enemy wanted me to do. I was in the battle of my life, trying to stay focused on God's promises for my healing. This woman was just one more arrow being thrown at me to derail my faith.

Sometimes we just have to declare, "Not today, devil!" If I had stopped, then the enemy would have won. I just stood my ground and prayed for God to intervene. Even though my flesh was a little afraid of what this woman would do, I continued to preach and ignore her. My refusal to allow the enemy to take any ground made her angry, and she eventually stomped out of the building. It wasn't until she stomped out that anyone else even noticed her. It was as if God was trying to show me that the enemy is really just an intimidator.

The devil wants to intimidate us into believing we are weak so he can get us to shrink back and wave the white flag of defeat. He is an intimidator, a terrorist who specializes in spreading fear and anxiety! His goal is to cause us to wilt in the face of opposition when issues arise in our lives. God wants us to know that in the face of fear we can look to Him as our rock and our strength. "Indeed, who is God besides the Lord? Who is a protector besides our God? The one true God gives me strength; he removes the obstacles in my way" (Ps. 18:31–32, NET). Be assured that whatever is in your way, no obstacle can stand up against the strength of God.

Look at the story of David and Goliath in 1 Samuel. "And the Philistine said to David, 'Come to me, and I will give your flesh to the birds of the air and the beasts of the field!'" (1 Sam. 17:44, NKJV). I love this account in the Bible because there is something so powerful about seeing someone inadequate make a comeback and overcome fear against all odds. Goliath was a giant who thought David was easy prey. David seemed so small in everyone's eyes. He appeared unequipped and inexperienced in warfare. Don't you love it when all odds are against us—*but God*! I will always root for the underdog.

No one knew that God had been preparing David in the secret place. Here was this big, strong giant trying to intimidate David by calling him names, threatening him with pain and suffering, and minimizing David's potential and value. This is the exact tactic Satan uses when he attacks us. He starts by intimidating us, telling us how small and weak and worthless we are. Then he calls us by every name that represents all of the failures of our past, making sure we know how ill-equipped we are in our own flesh. He will bring issues into our lives that cause pain and suffering and then attack our worth. All of this is designed to cause us to just give up, lay down, and quit, believing the lies.

Notice what David did. Despite what Goliath was saying, David stood up and ran toward the bully instead of running away from him. The Bible never said that David wasn't afraid. It merely states what he did in response to the enemy. Here is what David said to Goliath: "You come to me with sword, spear, and javelin, but I come to you in the name of the LORD of Heaven's Armies—the God of the armies of Israel, whom you have defied. Today the LORD will conquer you, and I will kill you and cut off your head" (1 Sam. 17:45–46, NLT).

Wow! David understood that he was smaller and weaker in his own flesh. So what did he do? He relied on the strength of the One who created him! Notice that David did not say he would defeat Goliath. He said God would defeat Goliath. David's response wasn't at all what Goliath expected. Rather than giving in to fear, David bravely declared his faith in God. As Goliath was spewing insults and threats, David ran out of patience and decided to get up and take action! Now is the time to stop trying to defeat the enemy in your own strength and start declaring to the enemy that God indeed has already won the battle! It is time to lose patience with the attack of the enemy.

GET UP AND FINISH THE RACE

I must be transparent here. I am not a very patient person. I get impatient probably more than I should. People who drive too slowly on the freeway truly frustrate me. People who walk too slowly at Disney World cause me great stress. People who stroll slowly in front of me while grocery shopping truly test my patience. To my way of thinking, there is no reason to stroll because there is too much to do. Listen, two-thirds of God's name is *go*! I am always on the go! I think I enjoy the beach so much because it forces me to slow down. However, when I'm not at the beach, I just want to scream, "For the love of productivity, just get moving! Honestly, do you not know the rapture could happen any moment? We're losing precious time here, folks!" Seriously though, I'm being a bit extreme here to illustrate how we tend to live our lives—impatiently. If that's you, then I'm pretty certain that like me your impatience catches up with you from time to time.

I remember one particular occasion when our son, Nate, was just around two years old. I was rushing through the grocery store, shopping for bread and grape juice for a communion service for our youth group. As usual I was in a hurry. There was a lady in front of me who seemed to want to read the label on every single item on the shelves (yes, I'm exaggerating, but it felt that way at the time). Every time I tried to go around her, she would position her grocery cart at an angle that made it impossible for me to get by her. In a moment of exasperation I leaned forward and whispered under my breath, "Lady, just move!" Well, as toddlers often do, my son decided to loudly repeat exactly what I had just said. He shouted, "Hey lady, my mom said, 'Just move.'" You can imagine my horror and embarrassment. I apologized as quickly as possible and moved on. There is a reason the Bible tells us patience is a virtue!

However, when it comes to the enemy, impatience is a good thing! Why? Because we are running our race, and the enemy wants to stop us. God wants us to finish strong. Fast or slow doesn't matter. We are to finish. The apostle Paul said, "I have fought the good fight, I have finished the race, I have kept the faith" (2 Tim. 4:7). I don't want to be a cross on the side of the road as a memorial to where I stopped before finishing my race.

Look with me at 2 Kings 6. A terrible situation was unfolding. The city of Samaria in Israel was surrounded by the Aramean army. It appeared that all hope was lost. There was no way to get food into or out of the city. "As a result, there was a great famine in the city. The siege lasted so long that a donkey's head sold for eighty pieces of silver, and a cup of dove's dung sold for five pieces of silver" (2 Kings 6:25, NLT). Do you see what fear caused these people to resort to? They were eating donkeys' heads and dove dung. Because of their stubbornness, donkeys symbolize mankind's tendency to do things in our own wisdom while the dove is a symbol of the Holy Spirit. The fact that they were eating dove dung could symbolize that they were living off of what was left over after the Holy Spirit had departed. Isn't that what we often do in crisis? We try to figure everything out in our own wisdom without the help of Holy Spirit, and we wonder where the power to defeat the enemy has gone.

Now, look what happened by 2 Kings 7. Elisha the prophet declared that by the next day everything would be OK! He spoke the word of God and declared God's truth over the situation. We need to surround ourselves with people who will prophesy the word of God over our families and declare, "It will be OK!" But that's not all that happened in this story. Let's look at what took place next.

> Now there were four men with leprosy at the entrance of the city gate. They said to each other, "Why stay here until we die? If we say, 'We'll go into the city'—the famine is there, and we will die. And if we stay here, we will die. So let's go over to the camp of the Arameans and surrender. If they spare us, we live; if they kill us, then we die."
>
> —2 Kings 7:3–4

Where are those who will declare, "Why sit here until we die?" Where are those who will not give up? Where are those who will get up and do something? In this story the whole city was paralyzed, crippled by fear of the enemy. As a result they were content to barely survive. It was a paralysis of analysis. The whole nation of Israel was paralyzed. It sounds a lot like our families when faced with crisis. We often sit back and analyze what is going on in the flesh while remaining frozen by fear, rage, and confusion. Revelation 3:2 tells us, "Wake up! Strengthen what remains." We must rise up and defeat the paralysis of analysis! "Get out of bed and get dressed! Don't loiter and linger, waiting until the very last minute. Dress yourselves in Christ, and be up and about!" (Rom. 13:14, MSG).

God wants us to get up, get dressed, and get moving when the enemy comes against us. Believe me, there were moments during my struggle with cancer when I got another bad report from the doctor and just wanted to throw my hands up and say, "Enough! I give up!" But then I would wake up, the light would come on, and God would gently remind me of the words of Psalm 18:28: "Suddenly God, you floodlight my life; I'm blazing with glory, God's glory! I smash the bands of marauders, I vault the highest fences" (MSG). God wants to wake you up by turning on the floodlight today!

I love this story in 2 Kings 7. Here are four guys with leprosy. The illness was causing their bodies to literally rot away. They were four outcasts, four guys who didn't fit in; they were diseased and contaminated and horrible to look at. Nobody wanted anything to do with them. They were just four dead men walking. Show me someone who has died to their flesh, and I'll show you someone God can use! Our flesh must die in God's presence in order "that no flesh should glory in His presence" (1 Cor. 1:29, NKJV). That means when God shows up, you need to get out of the way and let Him lead the battle. Can you see this? Everywhere these leprous men walked, they were dropping body parts. Then suddenly they have this crazy epiphany. One of them looks at the other and says, "Hey, we are going to die anyway, so why not get up and go visit the enemy? The enemy has food, and I'm hungry. Why not march right over to the enemy's camp and take our chances? What do we have to lose?"

We must get to the point where we are not willing to simply accept whatever the enemy dishes out. We must get to the point where we will trust God and move ahead in boldness and confidence that He will fight for us. God has already won every battle. These four guys were the forgotten misfits, the outcasts of society. They are reminders that God uses the ones no one would ever choose. The Bible says that early the next morning the four men got up and walked to the camp of the Arameans. When you decide to get up out of your fear, insecurity, complacency, and self-doubt and do something you never thought you could do, get ready because God will amplify your steps! Our steps are ordered of the Lord. When you are in a battle and God ordains your steps, the enemy will run, not you! And you had better believe the enemy won't be running toward you. God will amplify the steps of those who are simply obedient to get up and go.

> At dusk they got up and went to the camp of the Arameans. When they reached the edge of the camp, no one was there, for the Lord had caused the Arameans to hear the sound of chariots and horses and a great army, so that they said to one another, "Look, the king of Israel has hired the Hittite and Egyptian kings to attack us!" So they got up and fled in the dusk and abandoned their tents and their horses and donkeys. They left the camp as it was and ran for their lives.
>
> —2 KINGS 7:5–7

Don't you love how God brought confusion into the enemy's camp all because four forgotten misfits decided to just get up and go? By the time the lepers arrived at the camp, the enemy thought an entire army was marching on them. They didn't realize it was just four broken-down guys with leprosy. God was just waiting for someone to get up and get moving, and these four guys did. Are you ready to march forward, alone if you have to, in order to see victory? Perhaps you are reading this and you have relinquished your right to move forward. Somewhere along the way the enemy intimidated you, and you didn't get up and go. You didn't remember the battle has already been won. It's not too late for you to get back up. God is just waiting on you to quit giving up in life's battles right before the victory. Once you see that fear is just an aberration and a form of intimidation by the enemy, you can wake, get up, and move!

BRING THE VICTORY HOME

The lepers could have gone into the enemy's camp and taken all the spoils and plunder for themselves. After all, the city of Samaria had abandoned them, cast them aside, and written them off for dead. They could have left the city to starve. The sin of the religious is to believe that because you were hurt by the world, abandoned by people, and offended by society, you can just let them starve. But once we reach victory, we are not to keep it to ourselves. These four men did exactly what is expected of us when we receive victory over fear. Second Kings 7:8–9 tells us that as the four leprous men were enjoying the spoils of the victory, they realized it was wrong to keep it all to themselves. Even though they were cast aside, ignored, rejected, and abandoned, they went to tell everyone else in the city that the enemy was gone. They went into the city, knocked on the gate, and said, "We have won!"

These misfits, these outcasts, brought the victory home. Maybe your family has been talked about as if you are lost and without hope. Perhaps the enemy has isolated you and your family into thinking you are alone in this fight.

Or maybe the devil has terrorized your family to the point where you think there is nowhere to turn. If that is the case, then it's time to do something. It's time to prove the enemy wrong! It's time to quit allowing the devil to steal your freedom and cause you to doubt your worth. Stop allowing the enemy to bully you into a corner and put you in a prison of fear. God is waiting on you to get up out of the ashes and march into your destiny. You are a warrior who can send the enemy running into the shadows that once held you captive.

Stand up today and declare that you are a child of God and you are taking back your life and your freedom! Declare that you will walk in the power and authority given to you by God! Get up and get moving! It's time to awaken the warrior in you. Don't just sit there and let the enemy bully you. Remember, you are not alone in the fight. It's time to send fear into the enemy's camp. It's time for Satan to hear the army of the Lord marching with you! Ask God to lead the battle and then let Him help. Ephesians 6:13 says: "Be prepared. You're up against far more than you can handle on your own. Take all the help you can get, every weapon God has issued, so that when it's all over but the shouting you'll be on your feet" (MSG). Get up and raise your sword; remember whom you are fighting and whose battle it is. Remind yourself of what David declared when he battled Goliath: "All those gathered here will know that it is not by sword or spear that the LORD saves; for the battle is the LORD's, and he will give all of you into our hands" (1 Sam. 17:47).

I pray that you will find yourself up on your feet with a newfound strength and purpose, ready to face anything the enemy brings your way. I pray you hear the sound of a mighty army marching with you. I pray that fear has wilted as you realize whom the battle belongs to and who is fighting with you and for you. Get up and get moving today. The battle is won!

CHAPTER 11

HAVE YOUR DAY IN COURT

Be sober, be vigilant; because your adversary the devil, as a roaring lion, walketh about, seeking whom he may devour.
—1 PETER 5:8, KJV

Has the devil ever tried to throw the book at you? Maybe he has thrown all of your shortcomings as a spouse or a parent at you or kept you in fear that your family will fall apart or your children will fall away from God because you are not a good enough parent. Maybe Satan has accused you of being a mess in life and told you there is no restoration for you because you made your bed and now it's time to lie in it. Maybe the devil has convinced you God won't help you because you are reaping exactly what you deserve. The devil is quite the prosecutor, and he is skilled in his craft. He knows exactly what to say to back you into a corner of fear, self-doubt, and feelings of worthlessness. If you have ever found yourself in the enemy's twisted courtroom, then I (Karen) challenge you to call Satan out for who he is—a liar and accuser of the brethren (Rev. 12:10). If you are like me, you hate to be falsely accused. It just makes you angry. It is not acceptable.

The devil is the accuser of the brethren. He will come against us daily with accusations designed to wear us out and confuse us until we don't know what we believe. It's time we understand our adversary and his schemes. It's time we understand that Jesus is our defender. When we prepare our spirits by meeting daily with our Savior and studying the Word that has been given to us, we will be equipped to not only show up in court but to win! It's time to turn the tables on Satan and call him into the courtroom for a change.

First Peter 5:8 says, "Be sober, be vigilant; because your adversary the devil, as a roaring lion, walketh about, seeking whom he may devour" (KJV). I want to break this scripture down a little so we can understand what Peter is saying to us. The word translated "vigilant" is *grēgoreō* in the Greek, and it means to be on your guard, to be watchful, or to be attentive.[1] In other words, we must live with a watchful attitude toward the one who seeks to destroy us so no enemy or aggressor can be successful in gaining entry into our lives, families, or homes. Peter is stressing that we should *always* be on high alert to possible attacks of the enemy, not just occasionally. This means developing a lifestyle of continual, perpetual vigilance regarding the actions of the devil in our lives. We must make a commitment to deny the enemy access. This is the way we prevent the element of surprise the enemy is hoping to use to overtake us. Peter used the word *grēgoreō* to let us know that the devil is a shrewd, sneaky, vicious accuser and does not play fair.

The word translated "adversary" is *antidikos* in the Greek, and it is used to describe an opposing lawyer, a prosecutor who brings the accused to court and argues viciously against that person.[2] His goal is to win and then throw the accused in prison to rot away. That's the word Peter used to describe the devil. Peter is trying to tell us that when the devil accuses us, he often acts like a lawyer who brings us down by prosecuting us with lies or past failures that have been covered by the blood of Jesus. One of the devil's goals is to convince us we deserve punishment. If the devil is successful, we end up believing we deserve whatever situation is challenging us, be it sickness, financial difficulties, marital problems, or emotional pain.

The enemy wants to convince you that you are worthless and deserve to suffer. God on the other hand wants to show you that you are worth His Son's dying so you may have life and live more abundantly. It is unfortunate that Satan believes in our value more than we do. That is why he fights so hard to keep us blinded to it. Remember, God is our righteous judge. He has the final say, not the enemy. So bring your case into the throne room today and call the devil out! The Lord is the One who redeems your life from devastation, "who redeems your life from the pit and crowns you with love and compassion" (Ps. 103:4). Our God heals, delivers, restores, and redeems.

Have you ever heard a lion roar? Its roar can be so loud that it is deafening, causing fear and confusion. Satan's goal is to bring vicious attacks against your mind and heart to sow confusion and fear. His desire is to roar so long and loud that his accusations fill your mind to the point you can't hear anything but his lies. If you continually listen to the enemy's roar, he will eventually devour you and take you out. That is why it so important that we fill our minds, hearts, and spirits with the roar of the Word of God; the roar of the Lion of the Tribe of Judah is the loudest roar in the kingdom. God is the King of kings and Lord of lords. The enemy's roar becomes a cat's meow in God's presence. With all this in mind, let's paraphrase 1 Peter 5:8 in light of what we just learned: "You must be constantly alert and on your guard! The devil, a vicious prosecuting lawyer, will try to throw the book at you with lies and accusations. He is like a lion on the prowl—constantly walking around, roaring with a deafening sound to confuse you. He is earnestly seeking people he can catch off guard to devour!" But thanks be to God who leads us in His triumph!

GET BACK IN THE BATTLE

Not only are we to be on guard against the schemes and attacks of the enemy, but we are also called to resist him. James 4:7 says, "Submit yourselves, then, to God. Resist the devil, and he will flee from you." How do we resist the devil's accusations? First, we must submit to God. Then we must activate our faith. This requires going to a new level with God. I believe something is getting lost in the body of Christ. We have walked in fear and doubt for far too long. It is past time to sound the alarm and wake up to the next level! No more hitting the snooze buttons. We must wake up, activate our faith, and remain alert. I can get very intense about these things. In fact I care about you enough to say, "Get back in the battle!" It's time to grow up in your walk with God. It's time to use the authority that was given to you on the cross to call the accuser into court today. It's time to start believing what God says is true and just; God's Word does not change based on your circumstances or your moods.

C. S. Lewis said it best: "Faith…is the art of holding on to things your reason has once accepted, in spite of your changing moods."[3] Can we take a journey to a new level today? Remember, every time you get ready to go to a new land, your flesh will scream you don't belong there! Don't listen to the flesh. God is waiting on you to get there. Paul wrote, "In addition to all this, take up the shield of faith, with which you can extinguish all the flaming arrows of the evil one" (Eph. 6:16). Did you catch that? Your faith will actually extinguish the flaming accusations the enemy shoots in your direction. Are you tired of walking in fear, worry, insecurity, and a lack of desire for more of Jesus? If so, get ready! There is a breakthrough on its way. Let faith—persistent faith—arise and freedom reign!

I believe we need persistent faith in the church again. Why? Because the enemy is wearing this generation out with emotional attacks that leave them too scared to fight. There has never been a more lethargic, weighed-down, angry-at-the-world, forsaken, "leave me alone; I'm scared; I'm mad at God; the church is worthless; I'm all alone; I have to get mine; God has forgotten me" spirit in a generation! God calls us to be like Gideon's army in Judges 8:4, fainting yet pursuing! We must start living according to 2 Corinthians 5:7—"by faith, not by sight"! Let's refuse to give up fighting for this generation. Let's refuse to believe the lie that there is no hope for the future. Our faith has been so attacked that there are cracks in our foundation. It's time to fix those cracks so that we can stand firm. Our entire Christian walk is based on faith. Jesus is asking us today, "When did I stop being God?"

When we once again understand that it is through our faith that we are justified, then we will resist the accusations of the enemy. Romans 5:1–2 says, "Therefore, since we have been justified through faith, we have peace with God through our Lord Jesus Christ, through whom we have gained access by faith into this grace in which we now stand. And we boast in the hope of the glory of God." God is calling His people back to hope and authority, back to freedom and power, back to joy and purpose. He is calling us to action. He is calling us to declare, "No more sickness, no more lost finances, no more failure, accidents, or lost jobs!" No, "the righteous will live by faith" (Rom. 1:17).

Faith is about motives and motivation. So what happens when you don't see the progress of your faith? Can you still worship? Yes, of course you can—because of God's promise, not your progress. Sometimes we have to rely on the promise that God gave. Sometimes that seems like all we have in the moment. It's not about the progress we see with our natural eyes. You may feel as if you are walking in circles, but if you are walking in God's circles and if you stay right beside Him, you will see the promise fulfilled in His time!

"YOUR WILL BE DONE ON EARTH
AS IT IS IN HEAVEN"

Are you afraid to call the devil into court because you are afraid to appeal your case before the judge? It's time to approach the courtroom with confidence, boldness, and persistence to lay hold of your promises. When you were a child or a teenager, did you ever drive your parents crazy to get something you desperately wanted? You asked over and over and over even though you knew the limit. There was a line you knew not to cross. When you came close to that place, you would let up for a while, then start up again in relentless pursuit of what you wanted. That is called persistence. In God's kingdom persistence can be the key to the miracle. So many times we ask God for something, and when we don't get our way or what we want, we get angry! God is not moved by our temper tantrums. He is not persuaded by our childish fits. He is not our Santa Claus or a government bailout check. He is God. He wants to bless us, but first our foundation must be in place.

We cannot twist God's arm to get Him to comply with our wishes just because our flesh screams for our own desires. James asked, "What causes fights and quarrels among you? Don't they come from your desires that battle within you? You desire but do not have, so you kill. You covet but you cannot get what you want, so you quarrel and fight. You do not have because you do not ask God. When you ask, you do not receive, because you ask with wrong motives, that you may spend what you get on your pleasures" (Jas. 4:1–3). We have the right to approach the throne with confidence and boldness (Heb. 4:16). However, we need the right motives in doing so. We need to make sure that what we are contending for and being persistent about actually lines up with God's will and His way. We must understand that God's timing is perfect; just because we don't receive our breakthrough when we want or expect it does not mean God does not have a plan.

God's ways are perfect, "and we know that God causes everything to work together for the good of those who love God and are called according to his purpose for them" (Rom. 8:28, NLT). If we truly trust God and believe in faith that He hears our cries for help, then we know that everything we are going through will work toward our good, no matter what the plans of the enemy are. Know this: no one around you has the power to nullify God's plans. No one can steal the plans God has for you. No one can silence the roar of God over your life. The enemy can certainly cause the noise around you and the accusations in the courtroom to distract you from God's purpose for you, but the devil does not have the power to stop or change God's will.

You must make up your mind to keep your thoughts and heart in tune with God and be on guard at all times against the lies of the enemy. You can test those accusations against the Word of God to determine what is real and what is not, walking by faith and not by sight. Paul declared, "What if some were unfaithful? Will their unfaithfulness nullify God's faithfulness? Not at all! Let God be true, and every human being a liar. As it is written: 'So that you may be proved right when you speak and prevail when you judge'" (Rom. 3:3–4). Learn to walk in faith, without doubting, according to the Word of God.

WILL YOU CONTEND UNTIL...?

Walking through the cancer diagnosis taught us a very important truth about faith. Faith is incredibly easy to have until you are the one needing to experience it. It is so easy to tell others to believe and not doubt. It is easy until you find yourself waking up every single morning asking God to heal you. It is easy until you find yourself crying out for His healing every night when you lay your head down to rest. Then the questions become, Can I be patient in the waiting? Can I believe even when the doctor's report screams the opposite of God's promise?

There comes a point when your faith goes to another level and you rise up and declare that you *will* see the deliverance, the freedom, the healing, and the restoration you are asking for, no matter how long the war for that miracle takes in the heavenlies. God wants to know, Will you contend until...? As James 1:6 says, "When you ask, you must believe and not doubt, because the one who doubts is like a wave of the sea, blown and tossed by the wind."

Our faith, security, and hope cannot be dependent upon our emotions. If we walk according to our emotions, then we will be tossed back and forth and live a double-minded life. Our faith should be steadfast even when our circumstances seem unstable or shaken. It is about the *until*. I will believe *until* I see the salvation of my loved ones! I will believe *until* I see the healing miracle, *until* my finances are healed, *until* my children come home again! I will believe *until* fear is broken off my life! I will believe, not just for a day or a week or a month, and not just until I get tired of believing. I will believe *until* I see it! I will be persistent in my pursuit, persistent in my appeal, persistent in my approach to the King, and persistent in my faith!

It is time for a breakthrough! There is no more room for doubt. We must not allow our ruling to be overturned or overthrown by Satan in the courtroom. As Paul told the church at Ephesus:

> Finally, be strong in the Lord and in his mighty power. Put on the full armor of God, so that you can take your stand against the devil's schemes. For our struggle is not against flesh and blood, but against the rulers, against the authorities, against the powers of this dark world and against the spiritual forces of evil in the heavenly realms. Therefore put on the full armor of God, so that when the day of evil comes, you may be able to stand your ground, and after you have done everything, to stand.
>
> —EPHESIANS 6:10–13

HAVE YOUR DAY IN COURT

God is calling you to stand in His mighty power against the devil's schemes. The Greek word translated "stand" in Ephesians 6:11 and the end of verse 13 is *histēmi,* and it means "continue…to be of a steadfast mind…not waver."[4] We are to continue in faith and not be overthrown or demolished! How do we do this? We have our day in court!

We call the devil out! In faith we go to the edge of the light and take one step into the darkness. God wants to know, Are you ready for breakthrough today? Are you ready to go to another level in your battle today?

The definition of *breakthrough* is "an offensive military assault that penetrates and carries beyond a defensive line."[5] It is a forcible movement into a level not previously known. In other words, God is calling you to break into an area where you have not been before. We are not talking about gradual growth that comes with discipleship. We are talking about the place where you must go to get a miracle.

If you are going to break into a greater area of freedom, then you must continually push against your bondage and call the devil into court. Don't be afraid. Shout the Word at the enemy. "Cry aloud, spare not" (Isa 58:1, NKJV). This verse means to not hold back but to shout as if sounding a trumpet blast. We are to be bold when we call the devil to court! God wants to lead you into breakthrough. He wants you to put the devil on trial. It is time to fight! There are some things in life you will never get unless you are willing to fight for them.

Spiritual battles are conflicts that fight against our flesh. The battlefield is the place where forces define lines and engage. There are four spirits we must break through and defeat in the courtroom with faith. They are: the defeated spirit, the worried spirit, the poverty spirit, and the wounded spirit. Let's look at them individually.

1. The defeated spirit

This is a spirit that grows when we give up before the breakthrough, when the situation looks impossible, when we feel as if there is no way we can change things. We see it manifesting when we feel as if we have been overcome and it is time to give up, and we just begin to coexist with the issue we once believed we could overcome. Our nation is saturated with defeated spirits. We hand out condoms in schools for fear of teen pregnancies because doing so is easier than teaching values the world deems out of touch. We hand out clean needles instead helping people get free from addictions. The list goes on. We stop believing for the impossible and settle on mediocre as the norm, happy to have a dimly lit life instead of a fully lit life.

There is no room for darkness in God's presence. The Bible says, "This is the message we heard from Jesus and now declare to you: God is light, and there is no darkness in him at all" (1 John 1:5, NLT). The day of settling is over. It is time to get back what Satan stole from us. Perhaps you have been through so much you feel as if you will never win. We are too quick to take on the defeated spirit. Romans 8:4 says, "For those who live according to the flesh set their minds on the things of the flesh, but those who live according to the Spirit set their minds on the things of the Spirit" (ESV).

It is time to change your stance in the courtroom. God wants you to remember that "you will receive power [*dunamis*, the supernatural power for manifestations of miracles and wonders[6]] when the Holy Spirit comes on you" (Acts 1:8). Did you notice that there is no defeat in that scripture? There is power in your declaration and adoration of God. You can tell when someone is defeated by his or her vocabulary. Change your language and your vocabulary to be that of truth and praise and declaring God's Word. Proverbs 18:21 tells us, "Death and life are in the power of the tongue" (NKJV). Speak life! Speak truth! Speak hope! Speak love! And speak in faith! That's why Paul said in Philippians 4:8, "Finally, brothers, whatever things are true, whatever things are honest, whatever things are just, whatever things are pure, whatever things are lovely, whatever things are of good report, if there is any virtue, and if there is any praise, think on these things" (MEV). What we say reflects what we think. So no more stinkin' thinkin'! Allow the Holy Spirit to breathe new fire and passion and purpose into you today. When negative thoughts and lies of the enemy come in your mind, open the back door and show them out!

2. The worried spirit

I love this quote from Corrie ten Boom: "Faith sees the invisible, believes the unbelievable, and receives the impossible."[7] The opposite of faith is worry. Worry breaks the heart of God. God knows what we need and when we need it. In the Gospel of Matthew, God gives us a clear picture that shows He intends for us to live free from worry.

> Therefore I tell you, do not worry about your life, what you will eat or drink; or about your body, what you will wear. Is not life more than food, and the body more than clothes? Look at the birds of the air; they do not sow or reap or store away in barns, and yet your heavenly Father feeds them. Are you not much more valuable than they?

Can any one of you by worrying add a single hour to your life?

And why do you worry about clothes? See how the flowers of the field grow. They do not labor or spin. Yet I tell you that not even Solomon in all his splendor was dressed like one of these. If that is how God clothes the grass of the field, which is here today and tomorrow is thrown into the fire, will he not much more clothe you—you of little faith? So do not worry, saying, "What shall we eat?" or "What shall we drink?" or "What shall we wear?" For the pagans run after all these things, and your heavenly Father knows that you need them. But seek first his kingdom and his righteousness, and all these things will be given to you as well. Therefore do not worry about tomorrow, for tomorrow will worry about itself. Each day has enough trouble of its own.

—MATTHEW 6:25–34

God is not wagging His finger at us saying, "Oh, you foolish worriers. Don't you know?" He is a loving Father who provides so beautifully for His creation. "Look at the flowers of the field," He says, "and see how beautifully they reflect who I am. Yet they are nothing compared to you. Therefore, how much more will I provide for you?" God is our provider. We have no reason to worry! There will always be things to worry about, but as God's children we don't need to own the worry. God does the worrying for us.

It is time to kick the spirit of worry to the curb. God will pick it up and do with it what He intends. Let Him have it! We are the bride of Christ. What kind of a Bridegroom would let His beloved go through life weighed down by worries? Not Jesus! He calls us to seek first His kingdom and His righteousness, and as we do, *everything* we need will be given to us. We can walk upright, trusting in our Bridegroom day by day, and watch the accuser be reduced to a fumbling, bumbling nobody. Jesus said, "Make up your mind right now not to worry about it. I'll give you the words and wisdom that will reduce all your accusers to stammers and stutters" (Luke 21:15, MSG). The early twentieth-century evangelist Oswald Chambers is often quoted as saying, "Faith is deliberate confidence in the character of God whose ways you may not understand at the time."[8]

3. The poverty spirit

The poverty spirit is a demonic voice of fear! It says, "God doesn't have provision for you!" The poverty spirit opposes the goodness and blessings that God has for you. It is a mindset that can sneak in when times get tough. This spirit holds you down, creating a victim mentality that produces greed so you feel as if you deserve what everybody else has. It always causes a spirit of failure, removing all trust from God as you take matters into your own hands. A poverty spirit facilitates crime and fragments relationships, and it is always looking for someone to take advantage of because it feels defrauded.

It is easy to preach prosperity when everything is good and your bank account is overflowing with abundance. Then along comes the poverty spirit, devouring your resources until you begin to think you will never get ahead. Every time you do well financially, something else goes wrong. It is a constant swarm of locusts. The Word of God addresses such a spirit in Proverbs 3:9–10: "Honor the LORD with your possessions, and with the firstfruits of all your increase; so your barns will be filled with plenty" (NKJV).

There is only one way to defeat this spirit, and that is with the Word of God. Two scripture passages immediately come to mind to confront the lies of poverty the devil tells us: Matthew 6:19–21 and 2 Corinthians 9:6–10. Find them in your Bible. Read them often. Understand their meaning, and hold them close to your heart to use as weapons of warfare! Matthew 6 warns us not to store up treasures here on earth, telling us that God invites us to store them with Him in heaven because what we do in life has eternal value. We are to be rich in God, not the things of the world. How do we do that? Second Corinthians 9 tells us how—by sowing generously and reaping generously, giving for the joy and privilege of giving back to God with the same generosity He has toward us.

The poverty spirit does not mark those who don't have enough; it manifests in those who are driven by greed. When you are driven by greed, you never have enough. You can't enjoy what you have because you are always looking at what you don't have. Malachi 3:10 tells us to "bring all the tithes into the storehouse" (NKJV). When we obey this principle, God promises to open the windows of heaven over our heads and rebuke the hand of the devourer on our behalf (v. 11). Many are plagued with curses because they do not honor God in their tithes and offerings. Tithes and offerings are holy unto God. The word *holy* means separated or consecrated unto God.[9] Our tithing is not pleasing unto the Lord until we have the right attitude about it. Giving and using wisdom and common sense will break the spirit of poverty! By doing these things, "you will eat the fruit of your labor; blessing and prosperity will be yours" (Ps. 128:2).

4. The wounded spirit

The wounded spirit develops when we are hurt internally or carry around pain we haven't let Christ heal. When we experience emotional pain through tragedy, trauma, or disappointment, it can feel so real that it leads to a place of depression and despair. That's when we put up walls, fearful of being hurt again. Faith gets laid aside, fear takes over, and before you know it, you are paralyzed by fear! Proverbs identifies this condition, saying, "The human spirit can endure in sickness, but a crushed spirit who can bear?" (18:14) and, "A cheerful heart is good medicine, but a crushed spirit dries up the bones" (17:22).

Do you want to be vindicated and freed from the onslaught of the enemy's accusations today? Then go to court! When the enemy tries to wound you, it's time to get God's attention, not give up. When the heavens are silent, it is time to talk to God! Let's revisit how Jesus illustrated this kingdom principle.

> Then Jesus told his disciples a parable to show them that they should always pray and not give up. He said: "In a certain town there was a judge who neither feared God nor cared what people

thought. And there was a widow in that town who kept coming to him with the plea, 'Grant me justice against my adversary.'

"For some time he refused. But finally he said to himself, 'Even though I don't fear God or care what people think, yet because this widow keeps bothering me, I will see that she gets justice, so that she won't eventually come and attack me!'"

And the Lord said, "Listen to what the unjust judge says. And will not God bring about justice for his chosen ones, who cry out to him day and night? Will he keep putting them off? I tell you, he will see that they get justice, and quickly. However, when the Son of Man comes, will he find faith on the earth?"

—Luke 18:1–8

Wow! Can you see what is happening in this parable? The judicial system in the Roman Empire had its share of corruption. If you had money or knew someone influential, it could help your case with the judge. The woman in this parable was a widow. She had no money, no influence, and no husband. She was a woman with no rights. Yet she kept badgering the judge until he grew weary of her asking. Finally, in exasperation he granted her request just to shut her up. I love this! Her persistence led to her victory over her adversary, the one sent to torment her. The point of this parable is that if an evil and unrighteous judge will eventually give in to get a complaining, persistent, yet powerless woman off his back, then we can surely count on God, who loves us, to bring justice to our situations.

We can be assured that God hears us and responds in ways that are for our good. Our responsibility is to keep praying and petitioning the King. We must never give up! God hears us and He *will* respond. Even Jesus cried out with prayers and petitions to God. The Bible says, "During the days of Jesus' life on earth, he offered up prayers and petitions with fervent cries and tears to the one who could save him from death, and he was heard because of his reverent submission" (Heb. 5:7).

May I be transparent with you for a moment? When I received the diagnosis of leukemia, the devil tried on several occasions to bring me into the courtroom of lies. There were moments when the enemy tried to make me believe cancer would be my cross to bear, that I was just to do the best I could to live with it until the end. Sometimes when we don't see the answer we are looking for, we begin to justify our issue as just a test of our faith. I remember days when I would say, "God, if it is Your will for me to have cancer, then just give me the strength to make it to the end." Then one day as I was saying, "Even if You don't heal me, God, even if this mountain isn't moved, even if You don't part the waters, I still believe," God interrupted my doubt and set me straight.

All of a sudden the Holy Spirit quickened my spirit with a mighty inner roar of holy anger toward Satan, the accuser. The Spirit of God said, "No, Karen. This is a lie! Do not accept this!" Then God Himself gently spoke to my heart and said, "When did you stop believing I could move the mountain? When did you stop believing I could part the sea? When did you stop believing I am going to heal you, Karen? Do you trust Me?" In that moment I changed my stance and realized that court was indeed in session, and I was now the one with the righteous judge on my side. Losing was not an option. God said I could trust Him, and trust Him I would. There is no mountain God cannot move, no waters He cannot part, and definitely no cancer He cannot destroy.

Once again I petitioned God as one who knew the battle was already won. Taking hold of His Word, I cried out to Him with the words of the psalmist: "Listen, God! Please, pay attention! Can you make sense of these ramblings, my groans and cries? King-God, I need your help. Every morning you'll hear me at it again. Every morning I lay out the pieces of my life on your altar and watch for fire to descend" (Ps. 5:1–3, MSG). Every morning I cried out, "Every piece of my life! I will wait! I will watch! I will never give up and never accept the lies of the enemy. Your fire will descend! Healing will come!"

Whatever the enemy has brought against you—today, this week, this year, or whenever—you can receive your promises from God. Bring the enemy up on charges of tormenting a child of God. Call the enemy out and hold him in contempt of court. Are you tired of the enemy's constant harassment? If so, it's time for you to stand up, throw back your shoulders, and command him to leave in Jesus' name! Make up your mind to stay alert and watchful, constantly on your guard. You can be certain the enemy will try to come back to accuse you again. However, next time you will be ready for him!

Court is in session! The closing gavel is coming down, and the verdict is in. Satan will be thrown into the fiery pit, and we will win the battle. The righteous judge will hear your pleas for justice and mercy, and He will answer them!

CHAPTER 12

THIS IS YOUR NOW

For if you remain silent at this time, relief and
deliverance for the Jews will arise from another
place, but you and your father's family will
perish. And who knows but that you have come
to your royal position for such a time as this?

—ESTHER 4:14

Y OU WERE CREATED for more—more than just normal,
more than just average. You were created to expose and
thwart the plans of the enemy and lead others to freedom.
The way you see your value will determine your approach. It
is time to fulfill your purpose! You were created to do more
than fill space, more than just merely exist. Jesus declared
in Luke 19:13 that we are to "occupy" until His return (KJV).
To *occupy* means to move in and take control or possession
of something.[1] That doesn't mean we are renters, where the
enemy can come in and take what belongs to us. It means
we have ownership, and if we have ownership, we take and
protect the ground God has given us. We don't shrink back
or cower in a corner while the enemy takes possession. We

173

protect the land and our families from the enemy. Yet we cannot do this if we don't understand who we are in Christ and that we were created and destined for far greater things than the world has said we are qualified for.

Now that you know how to deal with fear, worry, and doubt, there is a question that must be answered: What will you do with the new freedom, boldness, and courage you have received? What will you do with your lionheart and your roar? You were rescued, revived, and restored for something greater than yourself. With great freedom and blessing comes great responsibility. God not only wants you to walk free of fear, but He also wants to see you rescue and revive both those around you and the next generation of freedom fighters. Your courage is so important in raising up a new generation equipped to keep the fire of God burning in the world. You are here for a purpose, and God has amazing plans for your life. Jeremiah 29:11 says, "'For I know the plans I have for you,' declares the LORD, 'plans to prosper you and not to harm you, plans to give you hope and a future.'" I hope you see how important and valuable you are!

Have you ever asked children what they want to be when they grow up? Many times they will say they want to be a football player, a firefighter, or an actor or actress. Many want to be a life-saving doctor or a judge or a lawyer fighting for those less fortunate. Some may even aspire to become president of the United States. But something happens as we grow older. Life somehow teaches us that we can only do what the world thinks we are capable or qualified to do. Maybe you feel as if you are limited or discounted because of the family you come from or don't come from, or because of how much money you have or don't have to accomplish your dreams.

Somewhere along the way someone perhaps told you that you are not good enough, not smart enough, or not attractive enough to be anything of value. Maybe you come from the wrong side of the tracks. One of the devil's biggest fears is that you will realize exactly who God created you to be and what you are capable of. The truth is God is no respecter of persons. As the apostle Peter put it, "It's God's own truth, nothing could be plainer: God plays no favorites! It makes no difference who you are or where you're from—if you want God and are ready to do as he says, the door is open" (Acts 10:34, MSG). God created this moment with you in mind!

It's time we answered God's roll call. Psalm 87:6 says, "GOD registers their names in his book: 'This one, this one, and this one—born again, right here'" (MSG). We must decide that at all costs we will not allow the next generation to speak of the last generation as a group that didn't want to see God's glory.

YOU WERE BORN FOR GREATNESS!

God is calling out for those who will stand up in the face of opposition and obstacles, who won't turn a blind eye to the attacks of the enemy. He is calling us to awaken to the cries of lost humanity, of the hurting and the innocent. He is calling us to confront the lost hope permeating a generation desperately in need of a God encounter. Will you answer God's call, or will you be one of those found standing on the sidelines, licking your wounds, whispering about your scars, and cowering in fear? It is time to step out of the shadows. We must declare, "Devil, you didn't make us, and you can't break us! We were born for greatness!" Your day of hiding is over. This chapter is for all the cave dwellers, those who are ready to come out of hiding. Alarms will go off in hell when you show up to get free. As the *I Am Remnant* manifesto declares, you are the remnant who "doesn't mind seclusion, knowing it is where strength is found, as [your] peace comes from secret encounters and private glances with the heavenly Father."[2]

I (Karen) want to take you on a journey into the life of Esther. She was someone God plucked from obscurity, from the wrong side of the tracks, and placed in a position of influence in order to bring about His will. Esther didn't know it, but her days of hiding were not to be forever because she was born for greatness. Her story is set against the backdrop of the Jews in exile in Persia. Carried there by King Nebuchadnezzar, they were under the rule of King Xerxes when the Book of Esther begins. Xerxes had everything a person could ever want. He was so wealthy that he threw a party for himself that lasted for 180 days. This was a guy who loved to show off the wealth and splendor of his kingdom. He was a braggart who boasted about everything that belonged to him, including his queen.

In the excitement of celebrating his wealth and power, King Xerxes called for Queen Vashti to come and stand on display so he could brag to all his guests. However, the queen refused to be paraded about.

On the seventh day, when King Xerxes was in high spirits from wine, he commanded the seven eunuchs who served him—Mehuman, Biztha, Harbona, Bigtha, Abagtha, Zethar and Karkas—to bring before him Queen Vashti, wearing her royal crown, in order to display her beauty to the people and nobles, for she was lovely to look at. But when the attendants delivered the king's command, Queen Vashti refused to come. Then the king became furious and burned with anger.

—ESTHER 1:10–12

Displeased and humiliated in front of his guests, the king banished Queen Vashti from his presence to make an example of her. It's easy to see why everyone was afraid of him.

As the wine and partying subsided, as it always does, King Xerxes realized he needed a queen by his side. The officials came up with a plan. They would search for the most beautiful girls in the kingdom, and the one who pleased the king the most would be made queen instead of Vashti. They said, "Therefore, if it pleases the king, let him issue a royal decree and let it be written in the laws of Persia and Media, which cannot be repealed, that Vashti is never again to enter the presence of King Xerxes. Also let the king give her royal position to someone else who is better than she" (Est. 1:19). The king liked their plan. He issued a royal decree that required beautiful virgin girls in the kingdom to be brought to the king's harem so he could choose his new queen. (Sounds a lot like one of today's reality TV shows, doesn't it?) By the sovereignty of God a beautiful orphan girl named Esther was among those young women.

> When the king's order and edict had been pro-
> claimed, many young women were brought to the
> citadel of Susa and put under the care of Hegai.
> Esther also was taken to the king's palace and
> entrusted to Hegai, who had charge of the harem.
> She pleased him and won his favor. Immediately
> he provided her with her beauty treatments and
> special food. He assigned to her seven female
> attendants selected from the king's palace and
> moved her and her attendants into the best place
> in the harem.
>
> —ESTHER 2:8–9

Esther was a Jewish girl who had been raised by her cousin Mordecai. When Esther entered the king's harem, Mordecai told her to keep her Jewish identity a secret because it wasn't safe to be Jewish in King Xerxes' kingdom. She and the other Jews were living in exile, as they had been brought into the land as spoils of war. They were a hated people group and victims of racism. It was a rough life for the Jews. When Esther walked into a room, people looked at her differently because she had no pedigree.

She was discounted and despised and had every reason to live in fear and insecurity. Both her parents had died, leaving her an orphan under the care of Mordecai. You can imagine she was a bit insecure. With no father to call her a princess and a champion like Pat does for our daughter, Abby, and no mother to show her how to make herself look beautiful and live as a strong, confident young woman, she just had to figure it out on her own. But at the same time, Esther was a Jew, one of God's chosen people. God wants you to know that you too are one of His chosen, and He chooses you today! He chooses you!

When Esther heard the king's decree, I'm sure she thought she didn't have a chance. Maybe she was walking through the city when the announcement was made. Maybe she was just picking up some food for Mordecai at the market that day. Can you just imagine her walking through the marketplace, seeing all the other girls from families of influence, prestige, money, and power getting their hair and nails done at the finest salons and saying yes to the perfect dress at the finest dress shops? They were all preparing themselves to be the most beautiful young woman in the kingdom.

Every family wanted their daughter to be chosen. Having a daughter chosen as queen would secure the family's status in the kingdom and give them a seat at the king's table. How sad that we often think what is on the outside, what is in our bank account, or how many followers we have on social media is what God is looking for when He chooses to use someone to make history. God often chooses the one everyone else overlooks and dismisses. He will call you out when you feel like the least in your sphere of influence and give you the opportunity to make history in the middle of your normal!

I can see Esther thinking to herself that she had absolutely no chance of ever being noticed. After all she was the least qualified, the least prepared in the eyes of the society she lived in. Maybe you have felt disqualified since the start.

Maybe you feel as if you could never amount to anything because of where you come from, what you look like, who your family is, how much money you have, or your past mistakes. Maybe you feel as if your past mistakes make you unworthy to make a difference. That is a lie from the enemy. God has plans for you. This is your moment to make history.

God is awakening those the world considers unqualified and disqualified. He is awakening those who have been hidden in the shadows, too afraid to step up and move into their destiny. Consider the words of the apostle Paul:

> Brothers and sisters, think of what you were when you were called. Not many of you were wise by human standards; not many were influential; not many were of noble birth. But God chose the foolish things of the world to shame the wise; God chose the weak things of the world to shame the strong. God chose the lowly things of this world and the despised things—and the things that are not—to nullify the things that are.
> —1 CORINTHIANS 1:26–28

I wonder if Esther even gave the possibility of being the queen a second thought. We need to understand that God can use us if we are willing, if our ears are tuned in to hear His call.

A REMNANT CHOSEN BY GRACE

When Esther entered the king's palace, a man by the name of Hegai, one of the king's servants, immediately noticed Esther's beauty. He saw something no one else saw. Out of nowhere Esther was chosen to receive special treatment, even though she was a nobody! God can choose you too, right now, in the same way. As Romans 11:5 says, "So too, at the present time there is a remnant chosen by grace."

All of a sudden the time came for the new queen to be chosen. Esther was presented to King Xerxes, who was able to choose the next queen from among a multitude of young women.

> Now the king was attracted to Esther more than to any of the other women, and she won his favor and approval more than any of the other virgins. So he set a royal crown on her head and made her queen instead of Vashti. And the king gave a great banquet, Esther's banquet, for all his nobles and officials. He proclaimed a holiday throughout the provinces and distributed gifts with royal liberality.
>
> —ESTHER 2:17–18

Esther's life was completely changed in a moment. One moment she was an outcast, hiding her identity, and the next she was living the dream. God chose a fatherless and seemingly forgotten young woman. It happened so suddenly it could have gone straight to her head. She could have become selfish and forgotten where she came from. She could have thought the moment was all about her. Sometimes that happens when God elevates us quickly.

Then Mordecai uncovered a plot by two of the king's men to kill the king. Mordecai told Esther, who then told the king. With this knowledge the king had the two men killed. Things began looking up for Esther; life was good and comfortable. Esther had gone from the wrong side of the tracks to living in the palace. Listen to me! We must realize that where we are now is for a bigger purpose than where we have been! Our current circumstances are not our final destination. We are being set up for something bigger and greater. Hold on! You have not arrived yet. You are on a journey to freedom, and you are called to take as many people on that journey as you can. The apostle Paul wrote: "Brothers and sisters, I do not consider myself yet to have taken hold of it. But one thing I do: Forgetting what is behind and straining toward what is ahead, I press on toward the goal to win the prize for which God has called me heavenward in Christ Jesus" (Phil. 3:13–14). Reach toward what is ahead!

I was a late bloomer and spent a great deal of my early life in hiding—from conflict, from crowds, from the spotlight. I was scared to step up or step out, scared to speak up and speak out. The devil was attacking the very thing I would eventually use the most to bring glory to God— my voice! I spent the majority of my life feeling as though my voice did not matter or that people would not want to hear what I had to say. I felt inadequate and ill-equipped, as though I was not eloquent in speech. I would break out in hives if I had to stand in front of a crowd. The enemy kept me locked in a prison of fear for so many years until one day God called me out!

If you had told me when I was sixteen what I would be doing now, I wouldn't have believed you. If you had told me all those years ago that I would be leading other people to experience hope and freedom, I would have thought you were crazy, delivering mail to the wrong house! "Return to sender" would have been my response. If you had told me just five years ago that I would be helping others get free of fear and healed of cancer, I would have said, "No way!" But fortunately there are moments when your destiny ignores your perception of yourself. There are moments when God the Father says, "There is more to you than meets the eye, but for now I will blind everyone so that only I have your attention! For now I will keep you hidden until your time and your moment presents itself."

What we call hiddenness, God calls preparation. To be hidden by God is evidence of His love as a Father. God will hide in you what you consider the uninhabitable regions of life to prepare you for the stage He is having built for your voice. The psalmist proclaimed, "Lord, you are my secret hiding place, protecting me from these troubles, surrounding me with songs of gladness! Your joyous shouts of rescue release my breakthrough" (Ps. 32:7, TPT). The Lord is preparing to release your breakthrough.

BE AVAILABLE TO GOD

God is not looking for the most qualified, most anointed, or even the most gifted. He is looking for one thing—your availability. It's about availability! Will you be one who declares, "I was placed here for something more"? Your destiny cries out, "There is more!" God is looking for those whom everyone else has looked past.

> This is my life work: helping people understand
> and respond to this Message. It came as a sheer
> gift to me, a real surprise, God handling all the
> details. When it came to presenting the Message
> to people who had no background in God's way,
> I was the least qualified of any of the available
> Christians. God saw to it that I was equipped, but
> you can be sure that it had nothing to do with my
> natural abilities.
>
> —EPHESIANS 3:7–8, MSG

There will come a moment when your normal becomes yesterday's newspaper clippings! It's time to awaken the warrior within!

My greatest concern for the next generation is that we are busy creating a party atmosphere in our youth services while the threat of spiritual holocaust creeps at the door. Where are those who get offended at the thought of people going to hell? Where are those who can hear the cries of the lost and the weeping of the angels? Where are those who realize that the flattering communication of life coaches who have lost their appetite for altars is causing the church to fall asleep at their infomercials?

You must choose sides. Matthew 12:30 says: "This is war, and there is no neutral ground. If you're not on my side, you're the enemy; if you're not helping, you're making things worse" (MSG). We must become ones who will step up when those who were most qualified decide to lie down. We must step up when leaders would rather dumb down potential warriors with Christian slogans, shallow grace messages, and meaningless hype than arm them with the power to rise up and lead a Holy Spirit revolution of truth. Don't be among those who offer up the next generation to the god of this world. This generation is in need of sons and daughters of God who will get to heaven with nothing left to do. God is looking for believers who will realize we were born for something greater than ourselves.

Comfort can be the enemy of vision and purpose. This is exactly what began to transpire in Esther's life. She was so comfortable. All her suffering had turned to joy. Her family was blessed and taken care of. She could have stopped being available to God. But in the course of events King Xerxes elevated an evil man by the name of Haman. Now, Haman was not popular with the Jews because he hated them. Egotistical and narcissistic, Haman wanted to be honored throughout the kingdom, but when all the nobles were bowing down to him in obedience to the king's command, Mordecai refused to bow. You see, the Jews only bowed down to God. God is looking for those who will only bow to Him—not to culture, not to popular demand, and not to shifting moods.

Mordecai's refusal to bow to Haman made Haman furious. In a fit of rage he ran to King Xerxes, spouting his hatred.

> Then Haman said to King Xerxes, "There is a certain people dispersed among the peoples in all the provinces of your kingdom who keep themselves separate. Their customs are different from those of all other people, and they do not obey the king's laws; it is not in the king's best interest to

tolerate them. If it pleases the king, let a decree be issued to destroy them, and I will give ten thousand talents of silver to the king's administrators for the royal treasury."

So the king took his signet ring from his finger and gave it to Haman son of Hammedatha, the Agagite, the enemy of the Jews. "Keep the money," the king said to Haman, "and do with the people as you please."

—ESTHER 3:8–10

The king's men went throughout the land declaring all Jews must die on the thirteenth day of the twelfth month. There was to be a holocaust that would wipe out the Jewish people. It seemed there was no one in the land who would rise up and cry out against this abomination. We may comfort one another into thinking we are more "civilized" and not living in such brutal times. But what of abortion? Every day thousands of babies are killed because they are helpless and there are too few voices to speak for them, too few to defend them. We must rise up and protect the innocent and let our voices be heard. We must be Esthers who are willing and available to sound the alarm!

DON'T MISS YOUR MOMENT

By the time we get to Esther 4, all of the Jews, including Mordecai, were weeping and wailing. Mordecai was wearing sackcloth. When Esther heard that, she sent him clothes, but he refused to accept them. He sent word to her, telling her about the edict and saying, "Girl, you have to talk to the king!" In fear for her life, Esther hesitated and told Mordecai: "All the king's officials and the people of the royal provinces know that for any man or woman who approaches the king in the inner court without being summoned the king has but one law: that they be put to death unless the king extends the gold scepter to them and spares their lives. But thirty days have passed since I was called to go to the king" (Est. 4:11). She almost missed her moment! She forgot that what is happening to us isn't always about just us.

Mordecai responded, "Wake up, Esther, or you're going to be next." Why is it that we don't awaken to our "today" until our tomorrow is in danger? I love the way Revelation 3:2–3 (MSG) puts it:

> Up on your feet! Take a deep breath! Maybe there's life in you yet. But I wouldn't know it by looking at your busywork; nothing of God's work has been completed. Your condition is desperate. Think of the gift you once had in your hands, the Message you heard with your ears—grasp it again and turn back to God. If you pull the covers back over your head and sleep on, oblivious to God, I'll return when you least expect it, break into your life like a thief in the night.

We must get up and do something, get up and make a difference. We cannot be silent any longer. We must cast off fear to see something greater than what we have settled for. Biblical truth is under attack. Christians must wake up and stand firm.

You and I are not here by chance. We are not an oops or

an accident. You are more than what you have become. You are more than what others have said to you or about you. You are more than what you have believed about yourself. You were born for greatness and for purpose. According to Job 14:5, all of your days have been numbered. God has been planning this moment your entire life. David said, "You saw me before I was born. Every day of my life was recorded in your book. Every moment was laid out before a single day had passed" (Ps. 139:16, NLT). This is your now! I am again reminded of David, when he reached the front lines to deliver food to his brothers in battle. When he heard the roar of Goliath taunting God's chosen people in 1 Samuel 17:29, he declared, "Is there not a cause?" (KJV). God is crying out right now, "Where are those who will declare, 'Is there not a cause?' Where are those who will run into the fight?" Don't miss your moment!

Mordecai told Esther, "If you keep quiet at a time like this, deliverance and relief for the Jews will arise from some other place, but you and your relatives will die. Who knows if perhaps you were made queen for just such a time as this?" (Est. 4:14, NLT).

With those words ringing in her ears, Esther stepped into her moment with God.

> Then Esther sent this reply to Mordecai: "Go and gather together all the Jews of Susa and fast for me. Do not eat or drink for three days, night or day. My maids and I will do the same. And then, though it is against the law, I will go in to see the king. If I must die, I must die." So Mordecai went

away and did everything as Esther had ordered him.

—Esther 4:15–17, nlt

Don't you love this? This is the response we should have in the face of the enemy's attack. We live in such a culture of "look at me" that we sometimes find it difficult to look outside of what makes us comfortable. Esther refused to use this moment for a selfie. She was willing to look through the telescope at the big picture instead of the microscope of her own world. The Jews were about to be exterminated. She decided that her value to the people was worth her going before the king.

Your "now" is calling! Will you answer or simply stand idly by and lose more ground to hell? As I think on this, I am reminded of World War II when Hitler was occupying territory throughout Europe. In 1938 the British prime minister, Neville Chamberlain, along with the French premier, Édouard Daladier, and Italian dictator, Benito Mussolini, made a treaty with Hitler called the Munich Agreement. After the agreement Chamberlain went back to Britain and bragged that he had secured "peace with honour," saying, "I believe it is peace for our time." He had chosen to appease Hitler. Ironically, less than a year after the agreement, because of Hitler's continued aggression and his invasion of Poland, France and the United Kingdom declared war on Germany. The Munich Agreement was one of the greatest blunders in history.[3] We must not repeat history. We have begun to appease evil in our time by allowing the enemy to advance and start calling the shots. We must rise up!

Elie Wiesel rose up. This famous Holocaust survivor said, "We must take sides. Neutrality helps the oppressor, never the victim. Silence encourages the tormentor, never the tormented."[4] Martin Luther King Jr. said our lives begin to end the day we become silent about things that matter![5] It is your time to wake up! This is your moment! The King awaits! I declare that your door is open and it is time to petition the King! Do not let fear hold you back. Stand and break the curse of fear off of your family for generations to come. The door is open to you! The Lord declared in Revelation 3:8, "I know your deeds. See, I have placed before you an open door that no one can shut. I know that you have little strength, yet you have kept my word and have not denied my name."

Esther had a now moment! As a Jew she was staring into the face of death! Remember, the king did not know she was Jewish, and she had no idea how he would react when he found out. Yet even with her life in danger, she rose to her moment. Look at what happened when Esther put aside her fear and decided that everything she had walked through and everything that had happened to her was for something greater than herself.

On the third day Esther put on her royal robes and stood in the inner court of the palace, in front of the king's hall. The king was sitting on his royal throne in the hall, facing the entrance. When he saw Queen Esther standing in the court, he was pleased with her and held out to her the gold scepter that was in his hand. So Esther approached and touched the tip of the scepter.

Then the king asked, "What is it, Queen Esther? What is your request? Even up to half the kingdom, it will be given you."

—ESTHER 5:1–3

Esther replied, "If it pleases the king, would you and Haman come to a banquet I prepared?" Haman was summoned, and they went to the banquet. God will prepare a banquet for you in the presence of your enemies. (See Psalm 23:5.) Fast-forward to Esther chapter 7, and we find Haman's evil plan coming to light. The enemy was destroyed by the very thing he planned to use to destroy the Jews.

Just as the king returned from the palace garden to the banquet hall, Haman was falling on the couch where Esther was reclining. The king exclaimed, "Will he even molest the queen while she is with me in the house?"

As soon as the word left the king's mouth, they covered Haman's face. Then Harbona, one of the eunuchs attending the king, said, "A pole reaching to a height of fifty cubits stands by Haman's house. He had it set up for Mordecai, who spoke up to help the king."

The king said, "Impale him on it!" So they impaled Haman on the pole he had set up for Mordecai. Then the king's fury subsided.

—ESTHER 7:8–10

THE FIGHT IS FOR YOU AND THE GENERATIONS TO COME

God is preparing a banquet for you right in front of Satan. He wants you to expose the enemy and walk out your freedom so your victory can strengthen others. Your decision to walk out of the prison called fear gives permission to your family and all those who see your actions to walk in freedom as well. An entire nation was saved from destruction because Esther did not shrink back or make life about herself. She saw a purpose beyond her comfort zone and a cause beyond her fear.

I walked through a very difficult and uncertain season after receiving the cancer diagnosis. Satan wanted me to accept the lie of cancer over my life and give in easily. The devil thought I would be an easy kill—but God! God called me out. He reminded me this life is a privilege, and we are here for a purpose. He reminded me that what I walk through is a good indication of who I am called to. I had to decide to either lay down and wave the white flag of surrender or let courage arise, put on the armor God has given me, and fight—for myself, my children, and my children's children. God was calling me to fight for the generations to come, to show them that life is about more than just me. He wanted me to show them how much God loves us, that His Word is true and just, and that He is our Redeemer and Savior. He wanted to show us that the battle is not ours; it's God's, and He has never lost a fight yet.

God awakened courage in me to be a light and hope in the darkness that would lead others to their freedom. My healing is not just about me; it is about you too. Know this today—your life counts. Your life matters. Your freedom, your healing, and your purpose await you. It is time to wake up, hear God calling you today, and respond. Let the generations to come know freedom because of your courage and strength. I am calling you to rise up! The King is extending the scepter. He is calling you to come to the throne with your petition! You will give an account for your now.

James 4:8 says, "Come near to God and he will come near to you. Wash your hands, you sinners, and purify your hearts, you double-minded." Tell God what you desire. Make your petitions known. This is your moment; this is your now. This is your opportunity to change the very course of history for someone, or perhaps for many. This is your opportunity to see a revolution and revival take place in our nation. This is your moment to cast off fear. God is providing opportunity for you to see beyond yourself to a world that is lost and hurting and in need of a loving, healing, good, good Father who wants to restore their hope and life.

CHAPTER 13

IF THEY CAN, WE CAN

...the lion, the king of the jungle, who is afraid of no one.
—**PROVERBS 30:30, TPT**

THROUGHOUT HISTORY THERE have been defining moments that radically transformed the world, shaping the destiny of individuals and nations. Today we are living in one such moment. Each one of us must decide that regardless of the political or cultural pressures we will not shrink back. The delegitimizing of the church as a moral compass in society has led to a decline of moral absolutes. As the people of God we must have courage. The thing about courage is that it is often absent until the moment when you realize silence is no longer an option. C. S. Lewis wrote, "Courage is not simply *one* of the virtues, but the form of every virtue at the testing point."[1] The greatest enemy of truth is silence.

Fear has the ability to manipulate the truth in us and turn a promise from God into a doubt and turn a lie from the enemy into a perceived truth. D. L. Moody once said, "To fear is to have more faith in your antagonist than in

Christ."[2] When you accept fear, it will turn your dwelling place into a room of scoffers. What do I (Pat) mean? When you operate under fear, you will find yourself sitting with those who appease your fear. This is why we must have a secret place with the Lord to hear what He is saying. We must always allow God to reinforce our virtues and purpose even while the noise of others shouts, "We have lost the battle!" I have learned that the longer you are away from the place of encounter with God, the more satisfied you become with being normal.

Normal today is considered yesterday's debauchery. Normal tomorrow will most likely be next year's old-fashioned concepts. This is why every day you must talk to God before you engage with people. When you spend time with Jesus, you gain fresh strength to combat any lie the enemy places in front of you. Regardless of what the enemy throws your way, just keep your eyes on Jesus, the author and perfecter of your faith. In this way you can be His voice and not the enemy's parrot. Charity Virkler Kayembe, coauthor of *Hearing God Through Your Dreams*, wrote: "Bill Johnson...teaches that whatever we are conscious of we manifest. According to him, we always release the reality of the world of which we are most aware. So if we are cognizant of the atmosphere of Heaven, the peace of His presence, and Christ Himself, we can impart Him. We can radiate His life and release His power into our world."[3]

If we are going to face the forces of hell in the days ahead, we had better be able to impart heaven. There is a reason Jesus instructed us to pray, "Your will be done, on earth as it is in heaven" (Matt. 6:10). Never forget that Satan is a thief. He wants your peace.

Let me take you back to the beginning of this book when I shared the prophetic word God placed in my spirit in September of 2018.

> My people are perishing for lack of knowledge. They have lost their will to fight. Fear, exhaustion, and culture have taken their roar away. They must be awakened and realize they are called to be voices of truth that carry freedom in their hearts and fire in their spirits. Restore the roar! Tell my lions to roar once again!

That word from the Lord gave me fresh motivation to arise and roar again. He is calling you to arise and roar too! The question is, Are you ready? Will you roar? God is with you! It is said best in the Book of Job: "Think! Has a truly innocent person ever ended up on the scrap heap? Do genuinely upright people ever lose out in the end? It's my observation that those who plow evil and sow trouble reap evil and trouble. One breath from God and they fall apart, one blast of his anger and there's nothing left of them. The mighty lion, king of the beasts, roars mightily, but when he's toothless he's useless—no teeth, no prey—and the cubs wander off to fend for themselves" (4:7–11, MSG).

DON'T BE TIMID!

The timing of your birth was not haphazard. God knew exactly when He needed you on the earth to roar for Him.

Yet roaring is not for the faint of heart. Our friend Dr. Michael Brown says it takes "thick skin, pure hearts, and steel backbones" to roar for God. It also requires a deep level of prayer and a keen ability to discern the voice of God. Not only will you be required to be brave, but you will also have to be loud. Now is the time for the righteous to "shout with the voice of a trumpet blast. Shout aloud! Don't be timid" (Isa. 58:1, NLT). We have the Joshua 1:9 promise: "Have I not commanded you? Be strong and courageous. Do not be afraid; do not be discouraged, for the LORD your God will be with you wherever you go." So I say, "Arise, lions, and defend the cubs of today. History is never made by those who choose to sit out the fight but by those who are willing to relinquish their fear and stand their ground against evil." Winston Churchill, British prime minister during the darkness of World War II, is often quoted as saying, "Courage is rightly esteemed the first of human qualities, because, as has been said, it is the quality that guarantees all the others."[4] No matter what comes your way, you must always remember that "we can confidently say, 'The Lord is my helper; I will not fear; what can man do to me'" (Heb. 13:6, ESV).

Your courage now will determine others' freedom later. What you are not willing to confront today will be the new normal for your children tomorrow. How you handle defeating fear today could be the doorway to someone else's God encounter tomorrow. There are stories throughout the Bible of those who grabbed hold of courage in difficult times. I am reminded of a powerful story in the Old Testament. This story is well-known, but there is one aspect of the story that captured my attention. It is the story of a group of priests who decided to confront a king. This king was very famous and feared throughout the land. His name was King Uzziah. He came to the throne at the age of sixteen. However, his beginning was much better than his ending. The Bible says, "He sought God during the days of Zechariah, who instructed him in the fear of God. As long as he sought the LORD, God gave him success" (2 Chron. 26:5).

Success doesn't make you; it reveals you. All too often, when people become powerful, they become full of pride. Such was the case with King Uzziah: "But after Uzziah became powerful, his pride led to his downfall. He was unfaithful to the LORD his God, and entered the temple of the LORD to burn incense on the altar of incense. Azariah the priest with eighty other courageous priests of the LORD followed him in" (2 Chron. 26:16–17).

King Uzziah was breaking the law by trying to offer a sacrifice on the altar. Only Azariah, the high priest, the one descended from Aaron, was allowed to burn incense on the altar. (See 1 Chronicles 6:49.) Here is the part of the story that receives very little attention. It says that Azariah and eighty other courageous priests followed King Uzziah into the holy of holies. "They confronted King Uzziah and said, 'It is not right for you, Uzziah, to burn incense to the LORD. That is for the priests, the descendants of Aaron, who have been consecrated to burn incense. Leave the sanctuary, for you have been unfaithful; and you will not be honored by the LORD God'" (2 Chron. 26:18). These priests could have stayed quiet. They could have enjoyed life. Out of fear they could have just looked the other way. After all this was the most powerful king in the world at that time. Instead they took a stand that would change the course of history. Never miss a moment to stand for God! If you will be His voice, then He will be the wind to carry the message.

GOD IS LOOKING FOR PRAYER WARRIORS

Who were those eighty courageous priests? We are not sure. We do know they understood that they had to do something regardless of the consequences. Azariah means "Jehovah has helped,"[5] and with Yahweh's help he became a catalyst for change. The eighty priests joined heart and soul with Azariah to confront an egregious act against the altar of the Lord. They did not flinch at the anger and tyranny of the blaspheming king. Instead they stood for righteousness, even though their stand could have cost them everything. We must learn from their act of solidarity. Together we can change the tide of culture.

Right now God is looking for bold and courageous leaders who have a holy fear of the Lord to arise and stand firm. These are those who are not worried about losing their reputations or their standing but understand that they gain strength and purpose in God. God is looking for those who will run fear out of their lives and homes by the simple act of living in a righteous manner. This means going against demonic forces, political winds, and cultural norms that fly in the face of God's Word.

Being one of these courageous leaders will require you to have a thick skin, a pure heart, and calloused knees from a life of prayer. But those who choose the path of righteous living will always be able to hold their heads up high, for they have established the deep understanding that "if God is for us, who can be against us?" (Rom. 8:31).

It is time to roar over the land God has given us. If fear has come into your dwelling place, then it is time to declare it has no authority over your family. Why? Because fear is the decapitator of your spiritual headship. Fear cuts off the spiritual head of the household to keep you from leading your family into their kingdom authority and prosperity.

For years Karen and I allowed the enemy to walk unabated into our home. Then one day dear spiritual parents, Pastor Al and Tava Brice, taught us how to pray correctly by coming into agreement with Matthew 18:19 and approaching God with our petitions. Our lives have never been the same since. They told us to always pray this passage from Philippians.

> Don't be pulled in different directions or worried about a thing. Be saturated in prayer throughout each day, offering your faith-filled requests before God with overflowing gratitude. Tell him every detail of your life, then God's wonderful peace that transcends human understanding, will make the answers known to you through Jesus Christ. So keep your thoughts continually fixed on all that is authentic and real, honorable and admirable, beautiful and respectful, pure and holy, merciful and kind. And fasten your thoughts on every glorious work of God, praising him always. Follow the example of all that we have imparted to you and the God of peace will be with you in all things.
> —PHILIPPIANS 4:6–9, TPT

Your family needs you to be courageous and focused. It is time to declare, "As for me and my house, we will serve the LORD" (Josh. 24:15, KJV). The fear of God is a righteous fear that will restore the land. God is looking for the courageous leaders who will rise up, march in, and say, "Enough is enough!"

WE MUST CONFRONT UNFAITHFULNESS!

The apostle Paul said that the greatest quality we must possess is being found faithful to God (1 Cor. 4:2). These faithful priests confronted the unfaithful King Uzziah. What happened when they did? Immediately Uzziah became angry. It's not hard to imagine that these priests thought they were about to die. After all this was the most powerful king in the world. In their flesh they probably wanted to run, but in their hearts they knew they must protect the holy place of God. The Bible says:

> Uzziah, who had a censer in his hand ready to burn incense, became angry. While he was raging at the priests in their presence before the incense altar in the LORD's temple, leprosy broke out on his forehead. When Azariah the chief priest and all the other priests looked at him, they saw that he had leprosy on his forehead, so they hurried him out. Indeed, he himself was eager to leave, because the LORD had afflicted him.
> —2 CHRONICLES 26:19–20

King Uzziah suffered from leprosy until he died. He was forced to live in a secluded place and never again went to the house of God (2 Chron. 26:21–22). His son, Jotham, took over the kingdom. Sadly, due to the significance of his father's behavior, Jotham never entered the temple during his reign (2 Chron. 27:2). His father's decision to be unfaithful caused his son to never again go into the presence of God. Unfaithfulness will cause separation from the place of intimacy! But the decisions of the courageous priests would lead to another person having a deep encounter with God.

According to tradition, the prophet Isaiah was the cousin of King Uzziah and his son, Jotham, who was twenty-five years old when he became king.[6] When King Uzziah died, it shook Isaiah's world. His king, his protector and hero, was now gone. The Bible ties Uzziah and Isaiah together in 2 Chronicles 26:22: "The other events of Uzziah's reign, from beginning to end, are recorded by the prophet Isaiah son of Amoz."

I truly believe that the actions of the courageous priests in the face of fear led to a young prophet having an encounter with God. Isaiah's encounter with God would lead to the roar of a lion and an Old Testament "upper room" experience. Isaiah was in hiding. He was seeking the Lord at a very dark time. What started as a funeral would lead to a spiritual awakening. The wail would become a roar! This is the promise of Amos 3:8: "The lion has roared—who will not fear? The Sovereign LORD has spoken—who can but prophesy?" If You will roar today, the next generation will see His face. Heaven opens when courage arises! The Book of Isaiah says:

In the year that King Uzziah died, I saw the Lord, high and exalted, seated on a throne; and the train of his robe filled the temple. Above him were seraphim, each with six wings: With two wings they covered their faces, with two they covered their feet, and with two they were flying. And they were calling to one another: "Holy, holy, holy is the LORD Almighty; the whole earth is full of his glory." At the sound of their voices the doorposts and thresholds shook and the temple was filled with smoke.

"Woe to me!" I cried. "I am ruined! For I am a man of unclean lips, and I live among a people of unclean lips, and my eyes have seen the King, the LORD Almighty."

Then one of the seraphim flew to me with a live coal in his hand, which he had taken with tongs from the altar. With it he touched my mouth and said, "See, this has touched your lips; your guilt is taken away and your sin atoned for."

Then I heard the voice of the Lord saying, "Whom shall I send? And who will go for us?"

And I said, "Here am I. Send me!

—ISAIAH 6:1–8

Restoration of the call happens when courage arises! What started as a season of confrontation, judgment, and sorrow would end with a young prophet encountering a mighty God and saying, "Send me, Lord!" That is what I call the restoring of the roar! God is still asking the same question today: "Who will go for Me?" Will you answer the call? Will you roar?

"Not called!" did you say?

"Not heard the call," I think you should say.

Put your ear down to the Bible, and hear Him bid you go and pull sinners out of the fire of sin. Put your ear down to the burdened, agonized heart of humanity, and listen to its pitiful wail for help. Go stand by the gates of hell, and hear the damned entreat you to go to their father's house and bid their brothers and sisters and servants and masters not to come there. Then look Christ in the face— whose mercy you have professed to obey—and tell Him whether you will join heart and soul and body and circumstances in the march to publish His mercy to the world.[7]

—WILLIAM BOOTH
FOUNDER, THE SALVATION ARMY

Keep God's love in your heart, and fear will never win. Choose to walk past fear and be an instrument for God, always remembering, "What, then, shall we say in response to these things? If God is for us, who can be against us?" (Rom. 8:31). This is your *now*. Release your roar!

Let's go change the world.

LOVE, PAT AND KAREN

P.S. What the enemy meant for bad, God turned for His good. (See Genesis 50:20.) Take that, stupid cancer!

APPENDIX

WE HAVE CONVERSATIONS with people on a regular basis who are battling some level of fear. As you are reading this today, do you feel as though your faith is wavering and trust is out of your reach? Do you feel as if life has been cruel to you and now you have to rely on yourself instead of God?

The power of God's unfailing love is infinitely greater than any attacks trying to threaten you. You can trust in Him at all times, as Proverbs 3:5–6 tells us to do. If we trust in riches or status or the ways of this world, our efforts will be futile. But God is our refuge; in Him our destiny is secure. In God our souls find rest and salvation!

Maybe fear has gripped your life so intensely that you can't think clearly. Maybe fear has caused you to isolate yourself, and you are sinking deeper and deeper and you wonder how to steer the ship back to safety. How do you begin to build past faith into a deeper trust? We talked about how trust requires relationship. Now is the perfect time to get to know the character of God and nurture that relationship with Him. Here are ten steps to get you on the right track:

1. Choose God and acknowledge Him. Romans 10:9–10 says, "If you declare with your mouth, 'Jesus is Lord,' and believe in your heart that God raised him from the dead, you will be saved. For it is with your heart that you believe and are justified, and it is with your mouth that you profess your faith and are saved." Take the first step and ask God to be the Lord of your life and start a new life.

2. Know God. Simply start a conversation with God. No rehearsed or memorized prayers, just you and God getting to know each other. James 4:8 says, "Draw near to God and He will draw near to you" (MEV). And we read in Psalm 9:10, "Those who know your name trust in you, for you, O LORD, do not abandon those who search for you" (NLT).

3. Read God's Word. Psalm 119:105 says, "Your word is a lamp to my feet and a light to my path" (MEV). God's Word is our GPS—God Positioning System—so we don't get lost on the journey.

4. Lean on God. Proverbs 3:5 says, "Trust in the LORD with all your heart and lean not

on your own understanding." Surrender control and let God lead you.

5. Praise God. Psalm 34:1 proclaims, "I will bless the LORD at all times; His praise will continually be in my mouth" (MEV). Praise opens the windows of heaven and creates an atmosphere where miracles take place.

6. Cry out to God. Psalm 61:2 declares, "From the ends of the earth, I cry to you for help when my heart is overwhelmed. Lead me to the towering rock of safety" (NLT). Make crying out to God your default against fear.

7. Listen for God to speak. Psalm 27:8 says, "My heart has heard you say, 'Come and talk with me.' And my heart responds, 'LORD, I am coming'" (NLT). Being a good listener is vital in building a trusting relationship. Simply respond by showing up for the conversation.

8. Let the Holy Spirit guide you. We read in John 14:26, "But the Counselor, the Holy Spirit, whom the Father will send in My name, will teach you everything and remind you of all that I told you" (MEV). Allow the Spirit to stir up your memory of all that God has done and how He has been consistent to His Word. The Holy Spirit is our spiritual compass.

9. Rest in God. Psalm 62:1–2 says, "Truly my soul finds rest in God; my salvation comes

from him. Truly he is my rock and my salvation; he is my fortress, I will never be shaken." When God becomes our fortress, there is rest for the weary.

10. Trust God. Jeremiah 17:7–8 declares, "But blessed are those who trust in the LORD and have made the LORD their hope and confidence. They are like trees planted along a riverbank, with roots that reach deep into the water. Such trees are not bothered by the heat or worried by long months of drought. Their leaves stay green, and they never stop producing fruit" (NLT).

NOTES

CHAPTER 1: RESTORE THE ROAR

1. This quote is widely attributed to Edmund Burke, including in a speech by John F. Kennedy, but it is more likely that this statement is derived from a quote by British philosopher John Stuart Mill, who said in an 1867 address at the University of St. Andrews: "Bad men need nothing more to compass their ends, than that good men should look on and do nothing." See "The Only Thing Necessary for the Triumph of Evil Is That Good Men Do Nothing," Quote Investigator, accessed April 8, 2019, https://quoteinvestigator.com/2010/12/04/good-men-do/.
2. Leonard Ravenhill, "What Is Your Vision?" (sermon, Calvary Commission, September 14, 1994), http://www.ravenhill.org/vision.htm.
3. George Scott Railton, *Commissioner Dowdle: The Saved Railway Guard and First Commissioner of the Salvation Army Promoted to Glory*, 2nd ed. (London: Salvation Army Book Department, 1912), 96.
4. "Let's Communicate," Lion ALERT, accessed April 8, 2019, http://lionalert.org/page/how_do_lions_communicate; see also Judith A. Rudnai, *The Social Life of the Lion* (Wallingford, PA: Washington Square East, 1973), 45.
5. Pat and Karen Schatzline, *Rebuilding the Altar* (Lake Mary, FL: Charisma House, 2016), 200.

CHAPTER 2: DO YOU TRUST ME?

1. Richard M. Langworth, "All the 'Quotes' Winston Churchill Never Said (2)," *Richard M. Langworth* (blog), November 16, 2018, https://richardlangworth.com/quotes-churchill-never-said-2.
2. *Merriam-Webster*, s.v. "faith," accessed April 8, 2019, https://www.merriam-webster.com/dictionary/faith.

3. *Merriam-Webster*, s.v. "trust," accessed April 8, 2019, https://www.merriam-webster.com/dictionary/trust.

CHAPTER 3: THE FORMULA FOR DEFEATING FEAR

1. Blue Letter Bible, s.v. "*dynamis*," accessed April 11, 2019, https://www.blueletterbible.org/lang/Lexicon/Lexicon.cfm?strongs=G1411&t=KJV. *Dynamis* is also transliterated *dunamis*.
2. *Merriam-Webster*, s.v. "dynamite," accessed April 11, 2019, https://www.merriam-webster.com/dictionary/dynamite.
3. Blue Letter Bible, s.v. "*dynamis*."
4. *Oxford English Dictionary*, s.v. "power," accessed April 11, 2019, https://en.oxforddictionaries.com/definition/us/power.
5. Blue Letter Bible, s.v. "*sōphronismos*," accessed April 11, 2019, https://www.blueletterbible.org/lang/lexicon/lexicon.cfm?Strongs=G4995&t=KJV; Blue Letter Bible, s.v. "*sōphrōn*," accessed April 11, 2019, https://www.blueletterbible.org/lang/Lexicon/lexicon.cfm?strongs=G4998&t=KJV.
6. Blue Letter Bible, s.v. "*sōzō*," accessed April 11, 2019, https://www.blueletterbible.org/lang/Lexicon/lexicon.cfm?strongs=G4982&t=KJV.
7. Blue Letter Bible, s.v. "*phrēn*," accessed April, 2019, https://www.blueletterbible.org/lang/Lexicon/lexicon.cfm?strongs=G5424&t=KJV.
8. These observations about the meaning of *sound mind* in 2 Timothy 1:7 are drawn from Rick Renner, "What Does It Mean to Have a Sound Mind?," Rick Renner Ministries, February 6, 2017, https://renner.org/what-does-it-mean-to-have-a-sound-mind/.

CHAPTER 4: WHEN THE SHADOW LOOMS

1. Elana Pearl Ben-Joseph, "Night Terrors," The Nemours Foundation, June 2017, http://kidshealth.org/parent/medical/sleep/terrors.html.

CHAPTER 5: JUST BREATHE

1. Blue Letter Bible, s.v. *"ruwach,"* accessed April 12, 2019, https://www.blueletterbible.org/lang/Lexicon/Lexicon. cfm?strongs=H7307&t=KJV.

2. Blue Letter Bible, s.v. *"pneuma,"* accessed April 12, 2019, https://www.blueletterbible.org/lang/Lexicon/Lexicon. cfm?strongs=G4151&t=KJV.

3. Blue Letter Bible, s.v. *"theopneustos,"* accessed April 12, 2019, https://www.blueletterbible.org/lang/Lexicon/Lexicon. cfm?strongs=G2315&t=KJV.

4. "What Is the Function of the Ribs?," IAC Publishing, LLC, accessed April 12, 2019, https://www.reference.com/science/ function-ribs-390a62c855c2627a.

CHAPTER 6: COURAGE, IT'S ME

1. Blue Letter Bible, s.v. *"Petros,"* accessed April 14, 2019, https://www.blueletterbible.org/lang/Lexicon/Lexicon. cfm?strongs=G4074&t=KJV.

2. F. L. Cross and E. A. Livingstone, eds., s.v. "Peter, St," *The Oxford Dictionary of the Christian Church* (Oxford: Oxford University Press, 2005), https://books.google.com/ books?id=fUqcAQAAQBAJ&q.

3. John Oakes, "What Is the Evidence That Peter Was Crucified Upside Down in Rome?," Evidence for Christianity, March 20, 2010, http://evidenceforchristianity.org/what-is-the- evidence-that-peter-was-crucified-upside-down-in-rome/.

4. James R. Sherman, *Rejection* (Cleveland, TN; Pathway Books, 1982); "We Cannot Go Back and Start Over, But We Can Begin Now, and Make a New Ending," Quote Investigator, accessed April 14, 2019, https:// quoteinvestigator.com/2015/11/05/new-ending/.

CHAPTER 8: LET YOUR PRAISE BE LOUDER THAN YOUR FEAR

1. Blue Letter Bible, s.v. *"diabolos,"* accessed April 15, 2019, https://www.blueletterbible.org/lang/Lexicon/Lexicon. cfm?strongs=G1228&t=KJV.

2. Blue Letter Bible, s.v. *"katēgoreō,"* accessed April 15, 2019, https://www.blueletterbible.org/lang/Lexicon/Lexicon. cfm?strongs=G2723&t=KJV.
3. StudyLight, s.v. "Entry for Strong's #2723—κατηγορέω," accessed April 15, 2019, https://www.studylight.org/lexicons/greek/2723.html.
4. Various versions of this list have been circulating for years. I heard Oral Roberts share a similar list years ago, but I have not been able to identify its origin.

CHAPTER 9: THE HIDDEN

1. Pat Schatzline, *Why Is God So Mad at Me?* (Lake Mary, FL: Charisma House, 2013), 62–63.
2. Blue Letter Bible, s.v. "Yĕhowyada`," accessed April 15, 2019, https://www.blueletterbible.org/lang/Lexicon/Lexicon. cfm?strongs=H3077&t=KJV.

CHAPTER 11: HAVE YOUR DAY IN COURT

1. Blue Letter Bible, s.v. *"grēgoreō,"* accessed April 16, 2019, https://www.blueletterbible.org/lang/Lexicon/Lexicon. cfm?strongs=G1127&t=KJV.
2. Blue Letter Bible, s.v. *"antidikos,"* accessed April 16, 2019, https://www.blueletterbible.org/lang/Lexicon/Lexicon. cfm?strongs=G476&t=KJV.
3. C. S. Lewis, *Mere Christianity* (New York: HarperCollins, 1980), 140.
4. Blue Letter Bible, s.v. *"histēmi,"* accessed April 16, 2019, https://www.blueletterbible.org/lang/Lexicon/Lexicon. cfm?strongs=G2476&t=KJV.
5. *Merriam-Webster,* s.v. "breakthrough," accessed April 3, 2019, https://www.merriam-webster.com/dictionary/breakthrough.
6. Blue Letter Bible, s.v. *"dynamis."*
7. Corrie ten Boom, *Jesus Is Victor* (Grand Rapids, MI: Revell, 1985), 184.
8. Harry Verploegh, ed., *The Oswald Chambers Devotional Reader* (Nashville: Oliver Nelson, 1990), 76.

9. *Oxford English Dictionary*, s.v. "holy," accessed April 16, 2019, https://en.oxforddictionaries.com/definition/holy.

CHAPTER 12: THIS IS YOUR NOW

1. *Merriam-Webster*, s.v. "occupy," accessed April 16, 2019, https://www.merriam-webster.com/dictionary/occupy.
2. Pat Schatzline, *I Am Remnant* (Lake Mary, FL: Charisma House, 2014), xx.
3. The Editors of Encyclopaedia Britannica, "Munich Agreement," *Encyclopaedia Britannica*, accessed April 17, 2019, https://www.britannica.com/event/Munich-Agreement.
4. Elie Wiesel, "Nobel Acceptance Speech," (speech, Oslo, December 10, 1986), http://eliewieselfoundation.org/elie-wiesel/nobelprizespeech/.
5. This statement is widely believed to be a quote by Dr. King, but it is actually a paraphrase of statements made in a sermon he gave on March 8, 1965, after civil rights protestors were attacked in Selma, Alabama, on the Edmund Pettus Bridge in an incident that came to be known as "Bloody Sunday." Dr. King actually said this: "A man dies when he refuses to stand up for that which is right. A man dies when he refuses to stand up for justice. A man dies when he refuses to take a stand for that which is true." See David Emery, "Did Martin Luther King Say 'Our Lives Begin to End the Day We Become Silent'?," Snopes Media Group, January 16, 2017, https://www.snopes.com/fact-check/mlk-our-lives-begin-to-end/.

CHAPTER 13: IF THEY CAN WE CAN

1. C. S. Lewis, *Screwtape Letters* (New York: HarperCollins, 1996), 161, https://www.amazon.com/Screwtape-Letters-C-S-Lewis/dp/0060652934.
2. D. L. Moody, *The Overcoming Life and Other Sermons* (New York: Fleming H. Revell Company, 1896), 12, https://books.google.com/books?id=i6HP-oJQBOoC.
3. Mark Virkler and Charity Virkler Kayembe, *Hearing God Through Your Dreams* (Shippensburg, PA: Destiny Image,

2016), 45, https://www.amazon.com/Hearing-Through-Your-Dreams-Understanding/dp/0768409977.

4. Winston S. Churchill, "Alfonso XIII," *Great Contemporaries, 1937* (London: Thornton Butterworth, 1939).

5. Blue Letter Bible, "'*Azaryah*," accessed April 17, 2019, https://www.blueletterbible.org/lang/Lexicon/Lexicon.cfm?strongs=H5838&t=KJV.

6. David Malick, "An Introduction to Isaiah," Bible.org, accessed April 3, 2019, https://bible.org/article/introduction-isaiah; see also Hebrew Nations, s.v. "Isaiah 1," accessed April 3, 2019, http://hebrewnations.com/articles/bible/isaiah/is1repent.html.

7. As quoted in Alvin Reid, *Evangelism Handbook: Spiritual, Intentional, Missional* (Nashville: B&H Publishing Group, 2009), 285, https://books.google.com/books?id=dh6RHGBlHrAC.

ABOUT THE AUTHORS
PAT AND KAREN SCHATZLINE

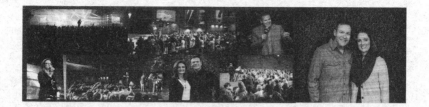

Pat and Karen Schatzline are international evangelists and authors. Together they lead Remnant Ministries International, an evangelistic ministry started in 1997 to call people of all ages back to an encounter with God. With a schedule that stays full year-round, Pat and Karen travel nationally and internationally, ministering a message of hope, purpose, and healing. They believe that now is the time for the remnant to arise from the ashes of defeat and step into their destiny.

They are the authors of several books: *Why Is God So Mad at Me?*, *I Am Remnant*, *Dehydrated*, *Unqualified*, and *Rebuilding the Altar*. They have written hundreds of articles that have been featured in magazines and on websites that are read around the world. Pat and Karen also have appeared many times on Christian television networks such as Daystar, GodTV, TBN, CTN, and JCTV, and on such TV programs as Sid Roth's *It's Supernatural!*, *Good News* with Evangelist Daniel Kolenda, and *The Jim Bakker Show*. Additionally, Karen is the host of a biweekly video blog called *The Breathing Room*, which reaches tens of thousands through Facebook Live and YouTube. The Schatzlines also enjoy being business owners and health coaches.

Pat and Karen reside near Fort Worth, Texas, with their daughter, Abigail. Their son, Nate, and daughter-in-law, Adrienne, are pastors of a thriving youth ministry in Modesto, California, and have made Pat and Karen grandparents of two adorable grandsons, Jackson and Anderson.

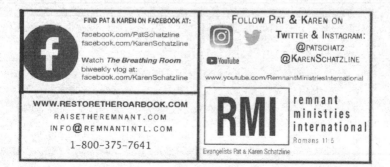

FIND PAT & KAREN ON FACEBOOK AT:

facebook.com/PatSchatzline
facebook.com/KarenSchatzline

Watch *The Breathing Room*
biweekly vlog at:
facebook.com/KarenSchatzline

FOLLOW PAT & KAREN ON

TWITTER & INSTAGRAM:
@PATSCHATZ
@KARENSCHATZLINE

YouTube
www.youtube.com/RemnantMinistriesInternational

WWW.RESTORETHEROARBOOK.COM
RAISETHEREMNANT.COM
INFO@REMNANTINTL.COM

1-800-375-7641

RMI
remnant
ministries
international
Romans 11:5
Evangelists Pat & Karen Schatzline

FEAR IS A DISTRACTION, NOT THE DESTINATION.

We are so happy you read our book. It's so important to expose and confront fear so that you can be courageous in your walk with God.

As our way of saying thank you, here are our **FREE GIFTS** to you:

- **E-book:** *I Am Remnant* by Pat Schatzline
- **E-book:** *Rebuilding the Altar* by Pat and Karen Schatzline
- **Printable Poster:** *Fear Not*

To get these **FREE GIFTS**, please go to:

www.schatzlinebooks.com/gift

Thanks again and God bless you,

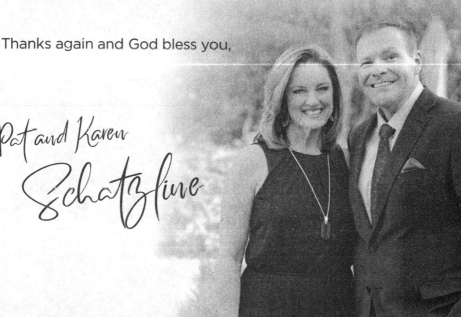

Pat and Karen
Schatzline

We know the spirit of fear is the foundation of the kingdom of darkness and the chief tool through which Satan works. Fear operates with the same principles of faith in a person's life. Simply put, fear is faith in the devil. To restore the roar is to restore faith. Pat and Karen masterfully give the reader the antidote for combating the spirit of fear, thus restoring the roar to the body of Christ. Fear doesn't stand a chance in the face of the Father's love.

—Dr. Scott S. Schatzline
Lead Pastor, Daystar Family Church

The formula for impact is the ability to do the right thing at the right time. *Restore the Roar* is the right word at the right time. Never before has the spirit of fear and intimidation so shackled the body of Christ. I believe that God has used Pat and Karen to share a message that will break these chains and release a roar of courage and victory in the lives of everyone blessed to read this book.

—George H. Sawyer
Co-pastor, Calvary Assembly, Decatur, Alabama

We are honored to endorse this latest book by Pat and Karen, *Restore the Roar.* You will be encouraged by their transparency and their track record that takes you to the only One who can deliver you from a spirit of fear—Jesus Christ! Many people do not realize how much fear is in their lives. In our culture today we have become experts at living with pain and masking our insecurities. Yet all the while, fear is affecting our thinking, our words, and our behavior, and all of this creates our character. May this book be a tool to help you find your way out of fear and into faith. It really does matter.

—PAUL AND KIM OWENS
SENIOR PASTORS, FRESH START CHURCH

Pat and Karen travel weekly across this nation and around the world; thus they have a unique perspective that allows them to identify universal issues within the modern church. As this amazing book reveals, fear may be the number one weapon the enemy uses to paralyze God's people. Thank you, Pat and Karen, for once again courageously exposing the enemy's tactics and offering biblical answers to this dilemma. This book will equip readers to face and conquer the fears that prevent them from seeing God's fullness released in their lives.

—RICHARD CRISCO
LEAD PASTOR, ROCHESTER CHRISTIAN CHURCH

All of us have experienced fear. As an emotion it is a good thing because it causes us to sidestep things that are intended to destroy us. As a spirit fear can be devastating to our faith. Pat and Karen Schatzline's new book, *Restore the Roar*, is sure to bring you face to face with your fears and cause your spirit to roar at the enemy! Before you finish reading this powerful book, you will hear the beep, beep, beep of God's delivery truck of grace backing up to the loading dock of your life to deliver your promise!

—DON AND SUSAN NORDIN
LEAD PASTORS, CT CHURCH

My good friends Pat and Karen Schatzline have done it again with this powerful book. *Restore the Roar* is a life-changing manual about how to shut the mouth of the enemy once and for all. Let these authoritative words encourage, inspire, and motivate you to overcome the fear and lies that threaten to destroy you.

—JAMIE JONES
LEAD PASTOR, TRINITY CHURCH

Both Pat and Karen carry the same intensity and resolve to see God's kingdom break into our realm. In *Restore the Roar* they are on a mission to raise up lions in the body of Christ who know their God. These are the ones with faces of lions, as those described in 1 Chronicles 12:8: "mighty men of valor, men trained for battle, who could handle shield and spear, whose faces were like the faces of lions, and were as swift as gazelles on the mountains" (NKJV). If we don't have the fighting spirit of the Lion of the tribe of Judah, Satan will be quick to snatch the truth away. In these times, we need to move with lions and be bold, to become people of exception, rising above societal norms and doing exceptional exploits in the name of Jesus!

—DAPHNE YANG
DEPUTY SENIOR PASTOR, CORNERSTONE COMMUNITY CHURCH

Since the beginning of time the enemy of our souls has utilized fear and intimidation to silence our mighty roar. Page after page of this book makes way for layers of fear to fall off. The reader's roar will be restored through powerful truths and divine revelation. There is no doubt that Pat and Karen Schatzline carry a strong anointing to deliver every reader from the spirit of fear and restore them to their God-given roar. If you have been bound to fear, expect to be set free!

—APOSTLE PATTY VALENZUELA
SENIOR PASTOR, IGNITE MOVEMENT CHURCH

Every believer in Christ has a roar that terrifies the kingdom of darkness. The attacks of the enemy are meant to weaken and eventually silence that roar. Through this book the Holy Spirit will awaken you and cause you to roar instead of retreat in the face of those attacks.

—JEREMIAH HOSFORD
LEAD PASTOR, ABUNDANT LIFE CHURCH

In a day when people are crippled by fear and doubt, I believe

God has given evangelists Pat and Karen Schatzline a remedy for this hour! Through this book I believe we will see a generation walk in courage, faith, and power. Let the overcomer arise!

—JAMES B. LEVESQUE
PASTOR, ENGAGING HEAVEN CHURCH

The power of the gospel is unleashed through the voice of God's people! That's why the enemy has worked overtime to silence you—he fears your voice. He knows when a righteous roar is released that devastates the works of the enemy and invites the kingdom of God into your trials, tests, and tribulations. My friend, through the pages of this book you will find your voice, be freed from fear, and release a sound that awakens the land!

—DANIEL K. NORRIS
AUTHOR AND PASTOR, GRACE WORLD OUTREACH CHURCH

Pat and Karen Schatzline's voices have been divinely chosen to be amplified to reach the lost and build believers. To be an arrow God uses to pierce the most hardened hearts is the greatest privilege anyone could ever have. If you apply the words in this book, this will become the experience of your life.

—FRANKIE MAZZAPICA
SENIOR PASTOR, CELEBRATION CHURCH OF THE WOODLANDS

I am so excited that Pat and Karen have been obedient to the Lord in writing *Restore the Roar*. Overcoming fear is one of the most needed messages in the body of Christ. Fear has buried more godly dreams than perhaps any other weapon of the enemy. I heartily endorse this book, both for its message and for the place of overcoming I know its authors stand in. Read and overcome!

—JIM POPE
SENIOR PASTOR, GRACE COVENANT CHURCH

As the child of pastors/missionaries and now a co-pastor alongside my husband, I have heard and even preached many messages on fear. None have impacted my life like this message from the Schatzlines. The truths in this book hit me with such power I nearly leaped out of my seat. Hope, faith, joy, courage, and the fire of God will overwhelm and change lives forever as a result of the Schatzlines' obedience!

—MIRIAM PHILLIPS
SENIOR ASSOCIATE PASTOR, RIVER OF LIFE CHURCH
JACKSONVILLE, NORTH CAROLINA

Restore the Roar inspires us to believe we were born for greatness. It will not only raise your faith to conquer fear and its crippling results, but it will also challenge you to a greater level of intimacy with Jesus and right living. Pat and Karen are transparent about how fear once dominated their individual lives and how they overcame that fear. Because of this victory they are tender and compassionate in communicating a biblical strategy for triumphing over fear. They skillfully develop the contrast between what Satan wants us to be—fearful, worthless, and deserving of suffering—and who our loving God says we are. He demonstrated our worth by sending His Son to die for us and now encourages us to trust Him, His Word, and His voice, not our circumstances. *Restore the Roar* is a masterpiece of encouragement to us all, and I highly recommend it. Lives will be transformed by this riveting and timely book.

—DR. DAVID GARCIA
EVANGELIST, MINISTRY128

Sometimes you open a book, and within the first twenty pages you realize it is touching the very depths of your soul. This is such a book! Pat and Karen Schatzline have written a book that doesn't just bring healing, but it also brings a newfound boldness to face our fears, and restore the roar.

—LEE MCFARLAND
PASTOR, LUMINATE CHURCH

In a word—wow! This book is a master class on absolutely

destroying any power that fear has in your life. It sets you up to tap into the unlimited reservoir of courage that has been so elusive. Pat and Karen Schatzline are incredible authors, having written several amazing and life-changing books. But in our view this is the book that has the most power to help so many people change the direction of their lives. We can't wait until we can put this book into the hands of everyone we care about. Thanks, Pat and Karen!

—Dan and Megan Valentine
Entrepreneurs and Life Coaches

This is a much-needed book for the twenty-first century. As we walk toward the purpose of God, we will face fear and worry, even as believers in Christ. Fear will create an atmosphere of loss and deviation from God's wonderful road map for our lives. When you read *Restore the Roar*, the Holy Spirit will encourage you prophetically. Pat and Karen wrote from their hearts. The anointing on this book will change your life forever.

—Rev. Louis R. Melo
Prophetic Minister, Louis Melo Ministries